# SPIRITUALIZING DIETETICS "VITARIANISM"
by Dr. Johnny Lovewisdom

# SPIRITUALIZING DIETETICS "VITARIANISM"

Written by DR. JOHNNY LOVEWISDOM, D.B.B., PSMC., MD, D.N.H., D.O.A., P.S.D., Ph.D., MS.D., S.S.D., T.O.C.

Doctor of Botanic Medicine, Naturopathy
and Osteopathy diplomas (England)
Doctor of Psychosomatic Medicine, and Hygienist-Dietician
diplomas (France)
Doctor of Psychology and Doctor of Philosophy degrees
(Spain)
Doctor of Metaphysics, and Doctor of Spiritual Science
(U.S.A.)

The last seven doctorates are from State authorized schools of the indicated nations. In 1966 Dr. Lovewisdom received the "HIPPOCRATES AWARD" given by the International Institute of Naturopathy (France) beside diplomas of Professor of Health, Professor of Natural Hygiene and Medicine. Professor of Human Sciences, while from the U.S. he also obtained a diploma as Professor of Natural Health.

Even greater were the achievements in the spiritual works, living the life of First Christian Hermits in a 13,000 ft. High Andes extinct volcano he became known to a hundred million people thru photo-illustrated magazine stories about the "Hermit, Saint of the Andes" in a seeming attempt to hide from the world. This was later followed with two of the longest fasts in history,-1953 completing 7 months 7 days and in 1954 achieving 6 months 17 days on 99% pure water, realized in California, only to suffer a veritable martyrdom when the medical authorities found out about it in 1955 being against all their laws of human nutritional necessities. He also has a degree in Philosophy for Yoga-Vedanta Forest University and has certified Tertiary of the Carmelite Order, the Oldest Christian religious order and of strict discipline also including the Essenes and "Sons of the Prophets" nearly a millennium before Christ's birth. Dr. Lovewisdom finally escaped from the grasp of civilization, now establishing his new project for the "Camp of the Saints" and "City of God" before the catastrophic World War III leaves another "Babylon" or "Rome" in ruin.

"The Lord God formed man of the dust of the ground, and breathed into his nostrils the BREATH OF LIFE; and man became a living soul." Genesis 2:7

"And God said, Behold, I have given EVERY HERB bearing seed upon the earth and all trees in which there is fruit of the trees yielding their seed, to be your food." Genesis 1:29

"And the Lord god planted a garden eastward in Eden; and there he put man whom he had formed. And out of the ground made the Lord God to grow every tree that is pleasant to the sight and good for food." Genesis 2:8,9

"And Lord God took man and put him into the PARADISE of pleasure to dress it, and keep it. And He COMMANDED him, saying: Of every tree of Paradise thou shalt eat; But of the tree of knowledge of Good and evil, thou shalt not eat. For in the day thou shalt eat of it thou shalt die. Genesis 2:15, 16,17

"THOU SHALT NOT KILL." "He that killeth an ox is as if he slew a man." Exodus 20 and Isaiah 66:3

"THOU SHALT NOT KILL." "All of you drink of this, for this is my blood of the new covenant, which is being shed for many unto the forgiveness of sins. But I say to you, I will not drink henceforth of this fruit of the vine, until I drink it new (Fresh) with you in the Kingdom of God." And Jesus said to them: "I am the bread of life: he that cometh to me shall not hunger; and he that believeth in me shall never thirst...He that believeth in me hath everlasting life...As the living Father hath sent men, and I live by the Father; so he that eateth me the same shall live by me...If any man keep my word, he shall not see death forever...

I am the way, the TRUTH and the LIFE." (The New Testament gospel of Christ) Verily God in Christ is "VITA" Life, besides the "VITA" way and the "VERITA-VERUM" truth. The truth is that we live by the Divine or CHRIST-VITA and the way is to be explained in the principles of "VITARIANISM." Those of the world still labor for flesh to eat and for their bread they sweat for this is their living, a living death, but we of the resurrection, restored to Paradise in the Celestial Kingdom live by Christ, who is Life Everlasting.

# CONTENTS

## LESSON 1 THE ORIGINAL DIET AND SIN

What has our Creator given as the perfect food for man? What is the most natural, good, pleasant to the eye and taste, food of Paradise? Why did man fall, how did man lose his original spiritual state, degrading to a creature fired with passion? The revelation of this is given in the Genesis and is the first law given to man about life on earth. It is the violation of this law that created the detestable Old Testament Bible history, and the sin of the world till this day, tho through its observation there would be realized man's return to Paradise. As much of the ordinary Bible translations are adulterated by explanatory additions and try to avoid rigorous discipline for the holy life, we have found that the Holy Bible of the Catholic version gives the clearest interpretation of the original scriptures in the light of spiritual perfection.

In Genesis 1:29 we find: "And God said: Behold I have given every herb bearing seed upon the earth and all trees that have in themselves seed of their own kind, to be your meat (food)." Behold here is the God-Given command as to man's perfect food. And also following this God's plan commanded there be a cultivation and reproduction of the fruit that man eats which is the purpose of the seed of fruits as well as the seed of herbs, and not that seeds should be man's food. Later you shall see that by participation in the seed of plants that God intended to be for the reproduction of them, instead of the herb and fruit alone, the deathless man of the perfect state comes to know death, after use of bread made of grains instead of the paradisical diet, his life is shortened to 125 years in Bible history besides commencing his journey in sorrow, passion for killing, lust of the flesh and painful existence.

Then in the second Chapter we are told that the Lord God (or Spirit) formed man out of the dust of the ground and breathed into his nostrils the breath of life, and man became a living soul (Spirit individualized). The Genesis is not a thing of the past but is on the Heavenly State of man and is eternally true. Today mystics are known to materialize more than one body (besides material objects) out of the elements of the atmosphere, just as the quickening Spirit in the beginning formed man from the dust which was activated by His breath or wind of wisdom to become living things. And then, "The Lord God took man and put him into the paradise of pleasures (Garden of Eden) to dress it and keep it. And he command-ed him, saying: "Of every tree of paradise thou shalt eat; But of the tree of knowledge of good and evil thou shalt not eat. For in what day so ever thou shalt eat of it thou shalt die the death."

Please note the word tree is again used just as before God states that man should "eat all trees that have in themselves seed of their own kind", which is obviously meant to be the fruit and not the tree, because man would not eat a tree. So eating the fruit giving knowledge of good and evil, or the fruit that gives virtue and vice, or the fruit of both spirituality and passion, man shall face death as his punishment.

Then later we are told how the man, both "male and fe-male", thru the work of God or Holy Spirit gave birth to another person without sexual or sensual reproduction, just as there are actually hospital cases often reported today of bisexual persons giving birth without sex contact, showing the eternal possibility of Paradisiacal or Heavenly Birth. Eve was formed of Adam of the neutral sex.

"Now the serpent was more subtle than any other beast of the earth which the Lord God had made. And he said to the woman: Why hath God commanded, "that you should not eat of every tree of Paradise?" The serpent even in the eastern literature is spoken of as spiritual fire, the "Kundalini", being the sublimated sex force which is materially seen in man by the form of the organ of evil, the only serpent that can speak and tempt. "And the woman answered him, saying: Of the fruit of the trees that are in paradise we do eat: but of the tree which is in the midst of Paradise (a garden :trees and plants or garden spoken or referred to as the edible fruits, and not the trees to be eaten), God said, Ye shall not eat of it, neither shall you touch it lest perhaps you die." The Pythagoreans intuitively knew this in prohibiting that the disciples pass thru a bean field lest they come in contact with the passion producing seed which God forbade the eating of. Why? Here is the sad result. "And the serpent said unto the woman, No you shalt not die the death. For God doth know that in what day soever you shalt eat thereof, your eyes shall be opened, and you shall be as gods, knowing good and evil. And the woman saw that the tree was good to eat, and fair to the eyes and delightful to behold and she took thereof and did eat, and gave to her husband who did eat. And the eyes of them both were opened and when they perceived themselves to be naked, they sewed together fig leaves and made aprons."

Yes, eternally and even today, if you eat the seeds of plants and trees, the forbidden food, tho they are palatable as Eve found, and make one wise, rather quick witted or brainy, one is tempted to have an eye-opening from the original innocence of the living soul. When living on fruit and herb, they were "naked and unashamed", but as soon as they chewed up, destroying the seed (material food in midst of fruit and herbs), this destruction of life in the seed, also created destruction of seed in men and women by seminal losses besides creating the evil to the eye so they had to cover up the lower organs excited by lust-producing food. To this day the serpent stands up in the lower part of the paradise of pleasures (garden of the senses) in man when tempted by woman, which cause in turn is original to the consuming of any seed, of herb, tree, animal or human (example: wheat, cashew nut, eggs or sex abuse) and results in man "knowing" woman, thus the fruit of knowledge taking woman to give birth by pain and man to toil with sweat on his brow till death takes them from their mundane misery.

I admit this nakedness of the truth may be an eye opener to the knowledge of good and evil, maybe our language may seem obscene and yet it is a true revelation as we can't beat around the bush of knowledge any longer leaving humanity to go to oblivion. Many times we may desire to do a thing, yet we try to justify actions that absolutely contribute against the effect we endeavor for. Using a passion and flesh producing diet renders one's efforts useless because at the same time one is feeding passion. People like to be "wise" as Eve tempted by the serpent, justifying sin as God-sanctioned by interpreting, "Be fruitful and multiply" in Genesis 1:29, as though it were a precept or first law commanded by God, when in truth as the Catholic Bible interprets it, this is a blessing rendering them fruitful because God had said the same words to the fish and birds, who were incapable of receiving a precept.

However, consider the need for this revelation in the world that so prays for the rest from desire, relief from pain, passion and plunder of nations. All sin goes back to the Original Sin when in eating other than the original diet of fruit and herbs, which gave us the burning fire of passions from which all sin is rooted. Nourishing from seed man generated more seed; becoming more passionate he less heeded the voice of God and took part in killing and other criminal sins. You know the story from there, how becoming a bread-eating people, they suffer in toil, give birth in pain, murder for a dish of lentils, kill to partake of animal carcasses, create war killing men to rob their cities, possessions, wives, children and so on.

There is an all sided meaning to interpret the Holy Scriptures, and before a statement can be used to show a symbolic truth, it should be illustrious and well understood as a literal truth as we attempted here. To achieve to the spiritual plane of life, we have to sublimate the grossness that makes one gravitate to the lower planes.

Stop now, before it is too late. Destroy the weed of temptation before it can grow into the history of sin described in the Old Testament. Give up the old Adam for the new Christ. The Adam and Christ ways of life have existed from the beginning of the world and accompany it to the end, and you are the one to decide whether man fails or becomes Life Regenerated.

"He who is naturally true to himself is one who without effort, hits upon what is right, and without thinking understands what he wants to know, whose life is easily and naturally in harmony with the moral law."-Tsesze.

"The serene, silent beauty of a holy life is the most powerful influence in this world, next to the might of the Spirit of God."-Pascal.

LESSON II
SIN-BIOLOGICALLY

That the "forbidden food" in the midst of fruits and herbs (Garden of Eden) is their seed, which if eaten destroys their own purpose of reproduction, and makes man and woman "go to seed", or approach death thru accelerating the egg production of the human body, besides stimulate the basic lower passion to which all other lusts are rooted, is the moral we hoped to present in the Genesis story in the "Genesis" of our course. Now we shall speak on the pathetic status of human society whose diet causes bodily sin biologically which has bearing on the moral, mental and spiritual life of man. Nor can we limit the Forbidden Food to seeds any more to include raw grains (the best egg producer according to poultrymen), raw nuts, legumes, and plant seeds in general, besides animal seeds (eggs), but all these have been modified to stimulate overeating by cooking, fermenting, spicing and supplemented by the products of animal slaughter to even more augment the fire of lust. Pleasures and production are looked for in human "egg mash" today.

No matter how we try to avoid it, there remains a mighty malefactor around that which the whole life of individuals is based, and which has only recently been brought out in our high schools where trouble is seriously manifest. They have boys' assembly separate from a girls' assembly in which they have speakers hint at the evil of what someone called "the great American sport" which certainly draws a stronger interest in lonely parked cars and in gang conversation than the respectable sports. Certainly in the past everything was done to keep the youngster's mind off of sex. Yet in spite of the absence of mental stimuli, sin was just as prevalent. If the body has been overfed on over-rich food, producing the typical fleshy American youth, nature soon sees fit to create a natural urge or "instinct" to make use of this excess flesh-making propensity. Youth curbs all his desires around this unique want giving the basis for a hurried family life. And if nature urges with all its power, it is only secondary that youth adapt his mental life and convictions into avenues that live in the sex. Is there a boy or a girl that reaches 21, becomes of age,-and still is a virgin? Yes, and those isolated cases only physically. How about mentally?

However, in the late teens youth does not have full access to sin to use up the continual flow of human seed that the over-fed body excessively manufactures, nor is it recommended that there should be, as the human population of the earth is already increasing too fast for its own safety, it is claimed. So, just like when your body is full of mucous from an excess of starch, it throws off the matter giving a clogged nose or other mucous discharge, so also is the excess seed substance lost through a really pathological discharge of menstruation or nocturnal emissions. It is this disease of civilization, this universal impurity of worldly people, and this status biologically in the original sin, that makes the human body biologically unfit as the "Temple of the Living God". It is also for this reason that the Holy Life could not be lived in a mixed society, but demanded the sexes be separated in hermit life monasteries, or other forms of asceticism.

Kindly notice we are presenting simple biological reasons for why sex life is sin, and not just basing our argument as it was preached in the past, on the holy scriptures. Nor are we going to make it too scientific and intellectual to elude the common understanding.

Why is it that a Yogi (Hindu devotee) is warned by his master never to touch a woman's body, that a woman at her time of menses is prohibited from public worship in the Brahman Temples and by some termed more poisonous than the cobra? Equally in the West, why do Christian monks have the same restrictions as to relations with the opposite sex, and why the strict separation in activities? This is not merely a religious superstition, but a biological concern in hygiene. In society it is called feminine hygiene, and covered up by using scents and perfumes that become a most effective base as male bait. It is the most poisonous in nature of the most foul smelling sin which expresses its gravity monthly in women, and continually in a lesser degree makes her the very magnet for sin continually. They speak of magnetism being a great factor in sensual love, but we doubt if this is a matter of magnetism so much as merely an unholy sex chemistry that she carries in her blood, perspiration, clothes, letters she writes and things she touches. Possibly it is the monk, the bachelor, and not the married man who is in contact with her, that most notices the "captivating scent" perceivable next to any woman and even things she touches, which immediately draws the mind to sex and sin. From this we may hint that the radiant worldly sensual love is only a smell that encourages appetite for sin.

In this study of the most universal sin whose catholicity can be seen in the fact that whenever you turn on the radio it most often blurts forth with an enticing "love" tune, beating even the next popular sport of killing and war stories, and is featured everywhere with pretty girls in advertisements, etc., this being the greatest attracting power in man's life, we need not encase all the blame on women. Please do not take our emphasizing with such gravity the status of sin in either man or woman as any reason for feeling hostile toward our speaking clearly, but realize we are offering a salvation from it, and before we can tell you, you should be cured, you must be convinced there is something seriously wrong to the point that you will be encouraged to do something about it. Woman is unconscious much of the time of her sin, even her ways of enticement being a second nature to her, but in men we find the deliberate intention manifest by his continual weakness to dream of far-off dance halls and other connections with women while he washes his car or at any other task, the continual interest in dirty stories and plain female worship.

Women are fortunate, their sin coming monthly, but nightly in cases, men have losses so that for their frequency they are called nocturnal emissions, if it does not get so bad as to be a continual loss thru the urine. Already in his teens, the male is a victim of a mild prostatitis. The lack of exercise in school life, the heavy constipating diet of bread, other starches, etc., create a pressure from the lower intestines on the prostate gland due to the only liquid intake being meat soup, etc., made of dissolving animal cell urine and no pure water. Every whiff of a female passing by, stimulates if not creates a slight ache so his brain is well conscious and fully aware of only thoughts connected with the organ of sin. Soon the glandular pressure becomes so great that even medically it is termed prostatitis, and the only temporary relief of the terrible rheumatic pain being immediate abuse, soon all manhood is lost giving the flabby, unambitious and well-aged man of forty only.

This sad status of civilized society seen in the popular divorce courts, embryo murder, contraceptives, sex bargaining, etc., sees not that "the children of the Resurrection shall not marry or be married." Marriage or "legalized prostitution" as someone emphatically named it because of ordinary practice, first makes it legal to sin all the way to Hell as long as it is with one person, and then if one is able to pay for another or more prostitutes one merely gets a government sanctioned divorce and license for new ones for greater sin. This they call a "scientific civilized world"! This is called an "enlightened Christianity"!-Barbarians and heathens! Puppets of Passion.

No, let us quit the evasion of truth. Where is the origin of sin,-spirit, mind or matter ? Certainly sin is not of the spirit of man for that is Divine. The mind of man is claimed culpable most commonly today, but could it be even reasonable to say that we sin by thinking! However, the mind is the product of the sense reactions, and we know the senses of the physical body are not reliable because they run after pleasures that too often result in painful results eventually. Matter, the opposite of Spirit or Truth, is the irreality and illusion. Flesh, whose evolution created the senses and the mind for its own protection, are all deluded by the transitory nature of matter.

They encourage the inexperienced starting in life that in masturbation the semen is waste of the body coming from the organ of excretion, that giving relief to the senses makes it necessary, and since it is a "natural" desire, it is as pure and holy as eating an apple. But is it? Or is the astrally provoked wet dream and menstruation as innocent and natural a function as it is defended to be?

By far, No! It is the curse on man for sin. It is the curse on man for his attachment to matter which makes his soul gravitate to earth and things thereof. It is a curse that cannot be done with merely by not thinking about it; it is rather due to thoughtlessness (not evil thoughts). How can one's mind dwell on spiritual things by force, and unconsciously live in sin? Yet it can be the partial cause in cases for splitting the personality into obsession and insanity. We have to be practical and master life omnilaterally on all planes. Tho it may appear we oppose monasticism, we do not, as it is good as far as it goes. It is unfortunate that in some instances the conflict of living a spiritual life mentally and having, in spite of it, sin manifest physically because of ignorance of a physiological law, has caused acts in monks and other religious people as severe as tearing out the organs of sin, but even at that, worldly people live much more insanely committing worse acts with no regard for morals.

The present trend to sex education, instead of hiding or ignoring it, is timely. We get no real results by being escapists in either avoiding evil thoughts or ignoring the matter. We must get down to the root cause of passion, face the reality.

Observing, we notice that fasting reduces the flow of menses and eliminates seminal losses. The great Christian technique for sainthood, or shall we call it "Christian Yoga", is based on "Prayer and Fasting". The Eastern technique is Breath Control and Mind Control, taught in 'Hatha' and 'Raja Yoga'. The Yogis have a postulate that absolute control of either the seminal energy, mental energy or the vital breath, controls the other two. That is, the Hatha yogi dominates sexual and mental energy thru breath control (Pranayama), and the Raja Yogi controls seminal energy and breath thru concentration. The Brahman Devotee or Yogi has a very old science of sex sublimation guiding the vital breath to energize the mystical centers of the body thru concentration; the Buddhist renunciate has a characteristic philosophy observing the abhorrent results of sin and the cause of such great and lasting suffering in their Nirvanic Contemplation, and the Christian saints in the prayers of religion visualize the perfect purity of the Holy Virgin in Meditation. The results are undeniable, -there have been some very great saints. But at this rate, not one in a million really lives the Perfect Holy Life, -when shall the Christ Kingdom be realized on earth? We have found the way simple, natural and effortless without forced breathing or forced discipline of the mind. Christ is trying to reach humanity in our teaching to give you the esoteric completeness of the way He taught for the realization of spiritual perfection.

But how do we naturally control the seminal force which appears to be the very nature of passion? Certainly we do not have the will power of Christian saints of the past, to be one in a million as I have said, to starve out sin from the body, measuring out 4 ounces of food for a meal once a day or fasting for days on end periodically. Nor has the Westerner the mental power of Yogis or other ascetics, his brain already with a loss of memory from the drugging of tobacco smoke, exhaust gases, etc., and with a thousand things towing his mind away from concentration. And likewise the other Eastern practice of breath control is impractical as his lungs are very weak having been cramped in the posture of indoor occupations and as we say burned out by corrosive air of cities instead of having vitalizing natural pure air since childhood.

However, there is something that the Western civilized man does best. That is EAT. This characterizes him all over, so let us start from there. The Western body thru hundreds of generations has become copious, we must remember, that is made for volume and also very efficient in taking a tremendous amount of poisons mixed with food. The European can take alcoholic drinks like water while the smallest amount that he gets away with, will intoxicate and injure the American Indian. What would happen if a multiple course dinner were forced into the Chinese coolie's birdsized stomach. However, with this ability is the cause of his being carried to an early death-he digs his grave with his teeth. So, not taking him from his most liked diversion, let us make a saint thru it: We mean controlling passion thru eating habits.

Our Lord God knew well what kind of lesson He had to teach man on earth, and it may, be for this lesson that He puts man on earth. Thus the first precept given to man in the Holy Book deals with what he should eat, and also tells him that disobedience in eating will cause his suffering and death as we told you in the first lesson. Next we shall show that man is physically composed of what he eats, and that the food characterizes the consumer's body.

That is real bliss which has no conditions; in the conditioned there can be no happiness; the Unconditioned alone is bliss; try to realize the Unconditioned (in thyself). Upanishads.

The great man is catholic minded and not one-sided. The common man is reverse. Confucius

LESSON III

FOOD CHARACTERIZES THE CONSUMER

"All philosophy in two words, -sustain but abstain", is attributed to Epictetus and this is the theme we apply in our way of perfection starting with the human body. The three foundations of the Christian Church, that is the three major teachings of Jesus's Sermon on the Mount, were ALMS GIVING, PRAYER, and FASTING. People pray because that is the easiest way to approach the Lord or to pretend Christianity. Some give alms with great expectations from this. Yet, who is Christian enough to use the complete key with fasting in it, so as to participate in the blessings of a whole-hearted love of God, undefeated Faith, the Holy Ghost, and healing of all physical ailments? Fasting is an essential for becoming a true Christian, for rebirth of body, and is the baptism of water that John the Baptist taught. Jesus declared it as an essential with the baptism of the Holy Spirit. Fasting was an important principle in the early Church, and is the greatest remedy of physical ailments, mental intranquillity and other barriers of spiritual discipline for the people of today.

Now all this goes to prove that what man eats is all wrong and too much. What has to be done is feed the body without poisoning and filling it with filth. We recommend the solution that Jesus gave as the immediate solution, that is, to make right one's ways by fasting to purify the body from disease and passion. However, we do not say one needs to live swinging on a pendulum from fasting to fasting constantly. Feed and fast at the same time: Feed the body enough to keep it strong, healthy, and vigorous, yet starving it of the impurities that bring on disease, passion and sin.

Now let us again look over our immediate general situation. Is the new generation of Americans a hopeless, inferior, unhealthy and dying race that may become extinct as some writers claim? With even women smoking, drinking and living recklessly, will our Western civilization end itself? No, not necessarily because evil has always had its origin in good, and the drastic status of things may shake the principles of its society into seeking something better. Realistically speaking, for the very reason of inheritance, the new generation has the greatest possibility for realizing a superior longevity because it is born with added resistance and adaptability. Is it the boy who has been healthy, strong and a great athlete that lives long enjoying life, usually? Perhaps you have noticed that not learning how to take extreme health measures in youth results in over-dissipation and ruin in the middle of life, while the weakling and experienced in disease early in youth is able to establish disciplining and health habits so as to make him often healthier after 60 than in his teens.

Also, all this terrible ruin of the nation's health in smoking, drinking and abominations in diet, may only be a change for the better in the new generation. Life is immortal and undefeated. There are obstacles, but it overcomes them generation to generation. Having need for adaptation, diseaseless plants and animals are bred to overcome the conditions that were adverse to them originally. We can say that necessity is thus the mother of adaptation in nature. Scientists say that at the ratio we are going, the human race will make itself extinct. Yet at the same time other scientists claim war is necessary to kill off the too rapid increase of population that threatens to make the earth's food production insufficient. Scientists only observe and support their sponsor. Let us go beyond appearances to the origin and cause of things.

However, we do not give the above as a defense for continuing the American way of diet, but conditions being as they are, they always have advantages to an optimist. Those who claim that the way man eats now is normal, support their argument by saying man is omnivorous. OMNIVOROUS is defined in the dictionary as "eating of all kinds of food indiscriminately, hence greedy", and that is the very thing Americans are accused of and yet seem to desire. Jesus warns against surfeiting and his gospel teaching of fasting is most pointed toward America. Americans have had their day, eating and drinking food products from all regions of the earth, wasting and destroying their abundance while elsewhere nations perish in famine. They realize not that by seeking pleasure at the disregard for suffering of others, in the end they have brought upon themselves envy, hatred and war. The omnivorous diet has developed the wild boar, hog, guinea pig, rat and civilized man into what they are, - selfish, inconsiderate of others, and miserable because of themselves.

Moreover the CARNIVOROUS diet, especially where other foods are abundant, is the height of sin. The youngster eating the hamburger or hot dog realizes not that while he is fattened enjoying all his appetites, he also is preparing himself for slaughter like a pig. Carnivorous feeding leads to cannon fodder. He who lives by the knife shall die by the knife. How can one expect to get a healthy living body out of dead putrefying carcasses of animals? He who lusts after flesh as food, also lusts after flesh in passion. Eating animals one becomes animal.

The same is true with other foods which characterizes the consumer. Universal and Divine Law is the most evident truth. He who lives on milk, a modification of the cow's blood intended only for a calf, becomes like the calves mother, that is cow-natured, cowardly or "cowy". Of course the nature of the cows may vary, though usually the dairy cow is well-sapped coward type. Just as mother's milk may change the nature of a child being modified by the endocrine secretions in the mother's blood from which milk is fabricated. In the case of goat milk the results are a goat nature. Eggs, the seed of fowls should not be considered any different from the hatched chicken that comes from the same substance. Animal seed is the most potent producer of human seed, raw egg being used to fortify abuse in sexual indulgences.

The diet of animal products is not only immoral, making man a killer and puppet of passion, but since the area for producing animal products such as butcher's meat is 16 times the area for producing a vegetable subsistence, it shows that he who eats meat and other animal food is "hogging" 15 extra acres of land for every acre he needs. With such economy is it any wonder there is not enough land for the people on earth to make a living and thus resort to war periodically to prune off the excess population? Each time you reach for that extra slice of meat, remember that you are cheating 15 men, or perhaps some poor peasant in the Orient, South America, war-torn Europe or our own city slums out of a number of bowls of rice, cabbage soup or bread.

The GRANIVOROUS diet is decidedly better than the two above mentioned diets because it is a notable fact that people who live on grains and are forbidden meat by religion or poverty, are of a peaceful nature. The Indians of the High Andes since the time of the Incas have been known for their pacifism. Also the oriental Indians, or Hindus who live on rice, millet, etc. are known for their peace-loving and nonviolent characteristics tho they are accused of needing birth control as the seed diet can be flesh producing.

Raw seeds and whole grains are really the most effective vegetable semen-producers, little understood by the present health-men who advocate seed diets for mineralizing the body. The seed diets certainly contain a good source of calcium, phosphorous, etc., for producing eggs in poultry, but we do not want to have the brains and nervous system of chickens? Tho seeds, nuts, grains, etc. have minerals needed in building brain, nerves, and bones, it is also a fact that they contain semen-producing properties which creates a continual overflow and loss of minerals from the body. The conservation of semen is like that of a dam, -if there is a regular small flow of water, the dam holds out, but continual overflow each time can tear it down to lose all the water already dammed up besides the extra amount that comes in. The well-fed American who has many times the food he needs, giving him many times the minerals ordinarily needed, because of its richness or semen-producing quality, it only goes down the sewer in menstruation, seminal losses, etc., and for this he pays in mineral deficiencies. The teeth are robbed of their minerals creating caries, besides bone degeneration, baldness, nervous trouble, insanity and disease in general.

I have come in contact with many interesting cases that conform to this revolutionary principle. Already when a boy in the teens, I was convinced man's perfect food should be fruit because eating fruit one causes no suffering to any creature nor does it even destroy a plant but actually helps the plant propagate thru the conveyance of the seed. Such logic naturally convinced me that the Creator has perfected fruit for man's unsurpassable solid food. However, then I refrained from vegetables because I reasoned that they get their nourishment from the soil and the crude inorganic matter from the soil is carried in the plant blood stream or sap, making the leaves, stem and roots grosser forms of nourishment. But unintelligently I used nuts as do the ordinary fruitarians who refer to nuts as a tree fruit. While traveling in a group throughout southern California in 1938, a former fruitarian presented a new concept contrary to the belief that nuts had a place in the fruit diet. He expressed It clearly, "Nuts make one nutty": And not only was this hilarious but a very true statement, proving to me by his telling me his own experience of being conducted to the "nut-house" through a diet of Brazil nuts and dates, but later I found numerous cases of the same mistake and result. People learning that fruit is a cleansing and nourishing article of diet, and decide to try it, only to get the opposite results because they mix in still a little heavy starches, nuts, or grains with the fruit. Sugar and starch, dieticians tell us, are the best mixtures for starting a brewery in the human intestinal tubing. Alcohol is made with a mash of potatoes, barley, corn, or other starches, which ferment with the addition of sugars. This may go on in the human intestinal tract giving spells of intoxication. Also the drawing of minerals from the brain and body cells caused by the protein and semen production from grains, nuts and legumes may thus create mental deficiency.

Not only did I begin to observe the numerous mental cases among the nut eaters, but also they were with defective teeth or toothless. A case of a vegetarian using nuts claimed he had nocturnal emissions every night. One can imagine the drain on the mineral substance from the brain, nerves, teeth and bones by this loss of the life concentrate in the semen. He soon lost his teeth in decay, besides becoming pathologically scatterbrained. A number of fruitarians I knew personally to eat nuts, avocados, or other heavy protein or seed foods have lost their teeth thru decay, because instead of bringing a cease of seminal losses, these foods make the losses even more prevalent, wasting away the essential tooth building materials. Certain South Sea Island people who never had any grains in their diet, though using plenty of sugar and starchy roots, have been found to have perfect teeth only until grains were introduced which resulted in rapid tooth degeneration. Anyone who has had bad teeth knows that a toothache can be relieved easiest by fasting and a cure for the ache permanently is abstaining from starchy mucous-forming food such as grains, nuts, and other starchy seeds. Not only is the starch-protein in grains, nuts and seeds a clogging mucous that stops up circulation of the blood vessels going to the teeth, but the protein actually robs the body of the minerals it already has thru stimulation of sexual losses of substance. Leaving the diet of Paradise consisting of fruit and herb man started the vicious cycle of worldly suffering, eating bread with sweat on his brow from labor. And the more he took in substance, the less he had, because the bread nourishing him temporarily, wasted away his body gradually till death overcomes him.   -

The HERBIVOROUS diet is the true way of mineral-izing the body. Herbs, including all the cultivated vegetables, contain a concentrated source of minerals (especially dehy-drated herbs, vegetables and seaweed). Yet they are without a toxic quality of protein which in the excess amount is convert-ed into uric acid that irritates the body cell chemistry causing so many aches and pains of the flesh, besides wasting away one's supply of essential minerals causing tooth, bone, brain and nerve degeneration. Instead of looking to the dog and cat, we should take a dietetic lesson from the elephant, horse and oxen as to how to build a mighty physique that will endure constant, heavy labor.

In summary, by the simple, sincere and astounding presentation of the truth on how food characterizes people we demonstrate Universal Law in Nature. The Omnivorous diet makes one rat-like and piggish. Our civilized cities are little more than a rat nest and hog pen, analyzing the amount of filth sold at eating places as food. Hog hogs hog and rat robs rat! Living on animal carcasses is the quickest way to become a carcass. The hamburger-fed is destined to become hamburg-er-spread in the battlefield. Living by killing, one soon dies by being killed. Egg eating may step up egg production but at a loss. Calves are raised from cow's milk. Tobacco, black coffee, and distilled alcohol produces a "dope living", a bitter and un-bearable existence. The "sour puss" is raised on an acid diet. A pasty complexion and cadaveric appearance is derived from pastry, bread and other white flour products or pastes. There is nothing like white flour paste, animal grease and glue for clogging up and putting the human mechanism out of com-mission. On the other hand, sweets make one sweet. Eating apples one becomes the apple of everyone's eye. If you will eat peaches, you will be peachy. (Really, no kidding!) Living on pure food (fruit and herbs) one becomes pure in body. Partak-ing fully in life one is full of life.

This is an entertaining besides serious way to look upon dietetics. Writers make us think we have to be specialists in medicine to be able to eat.

LESSON IV

## THE RETURN TO GOD-GIVEN FOOD

"Stop !" If you are living wrong, every action onward is conducting you into a worse calamity. This is what Nature exclaims in all sentient beings in danger. However, man, the dumbest animal (at least instinctively), long ago got rid of the "Stop" signal so he can go on in the wrong direction just as tranquil as ever...Animals and natural man, when sick lose their appetite and do not eat,-for days often,-but the civilized have appetizers, stimulants and other inventions to continue on the wrong road. Very few people are free of any kind of ailment. Very few people have an appetite for good natural food as God has given it to us. Are you hungry ever? Or do you just want to be stimulated. Most people are not at peace unless they have a habitual ferment of starches and sugars, the burning of meat's uric acid or of spices and salt, the lift-up of a cup of coffee, cigarettes and alcohol, not to speak of the stylish shot-in-the-arm and other medical props to make them "strong and alive". Yes, "strong and alive" chemically and bacteriologically! People eat because of the clock ("time to be hungry"), because if they don't they'll get weak and because the fire of artificial stimulation gives out.

We drown out the omnipresent intelligence of the Creator in Nature so we have to refer to a book to guide us in living. But what is the first thing that Jesus did when starting His teaching described in the New Testament? He took on the Baptism of penance and fasted 40 days with no food after which he hungered. This is very significant that He hungered only after 40 days and 40 nights without food. Most people never hunger. They only are victims of appetites and passion. Before one can be hungry in the real sense, one has to fast till hunger returns or when one can relish natural fruit and herb without artificial stimulants.

Now in the Christian Technique of Spiritual Attainment, or shall we name it "Christian Yoga", or the "Sainthood", what is the first teaching given by the Great Master? The first precept in the Old Testament was the eating of fruit and herb, and the first precept of the Saviour in the New Testament is again a reference to the God Given precept, or rather the penalty for its transgression. "......Jesus began to preach and to say: "Do penance for the Kingdom of Heaven is at hand." (Math. 4:17) Doing penance means fasting and Prayer, self-punishment for past errors. Again what does the Lord Christ say when He refers to the omnipotent key to Godhood, with which "Nothing will be impossible unto you" (Math. 17:20). This key, Faith to move mountains, or the God-Power, sustained only by "prayer and Fasting." Also we are well assured that "unless you shall do penance, you shall all likewise perish" (Luke 13:3,5). Most religionists are hoping for a heaven without effort. Rather they realize not that heaven is attained effortlessly without continual slavery to the whims of the senses and for recovery of substance.

One cannot fast too long, ever. Thru clinical experience, fasting experts have fasted people up to three months and claim there is no limit. The usual prescription of the rational fast until hunger returns, which is usually around 40 days depending on the condition that has to be renewed and regenerated. After forty days Jesus hungered.

Moreover, in Christ we shall neither hunger nor thirst (John 6:35). We are not to be solicitous as to our life, what we shall eat and drink for the Spiritual plane of life. A number of Christian mystics have attained to abstaining from food for life. Today's great example of total and perpetual abstinence is Theresa Neumann, Bavarian saint, who has not eaten since 1923 nor drank any liquid since 1927.

The main thing to remember is that fasting gives you omnipotence, i.e. "nothing shall be impossible unto you". For the man who lives on bread, meat and coffee three times a day to think of living on a few "flat insipid" fruits and a salad as a daily menu is unpleasant to contemplate. However, I do remember the first orange I ate after a forty day fast; I had never tasted such ecstasy out of merely eating and it was well worth 40 days for one orange so delicious yet available to anyone. The simple and natural diet becomes very appetizing and strengthening to a clean body after a fast. And the cleaner one is by fasting, the more godly one becomes.

As to instruction in fasting, one should know that it is not the fasting that is apt to be misunderstood, but rather it is the breaking of the fast that may either heal or kill you. The so-called deaths-from-starvation could have been avoided by correct fast-breaking procedure. After weeks of fasting the body is in no condition to receive heavy nourishment, the digestive juices are not active so that assimilation is poor or impossible and otherwise there is need of adjustment to return to food. First, one must cleanse the morbid matter away taking acid fruit juices, diluted in water, then after a couple days one can gradually go on fruit juice, fresh fruit and when one half the number of days of the fast is completed, one can gradually start on salads till one is back, to the desired diet. A forty day fast needs forty days weaning back to one's customary diet. People have killed themselves by going 20 or 30 days without food and then eating bread, potatoes, etc., pasting up their system so nothing could go thru the shrunken digestive channels. The most often used fruit juice is orange juice, but Nature will tell you just what is best in your true hunger, probably being some juicy fruit or berry in season. Jesus (according to certain Vatican scriptures) is said to have told people to fast one day for each year of abuse on a corrupt diet. That is, forty years of wrong living is amended by forty days of fasting, tho Jesus in spiritual purpose fasted that length of time when only 29 years old.

The fast will tone up the system so that foods will be very profitably assimilated and the vigor will come to that of youth in the teens. A correctly broken fast may even produce seminal losses if heavy protein foods are used which before did not provoke passion perhaps because of the new efficiency of assimilation and cell building potentiality.

A long fast may be enough to rid one of passion so that one can go right on the fruit and vegetable diet immediately. However, if the person is of a temperament that is unable to fast more than about 3 days to start with, then a "fruit fast" for seven months will surely heal one from passion and strengthen the organs for complete conservation of one's vital fluids.

Fresh fruits were given as a pleasing and adequate sustenance for man, and are a secure refuge for living free from
passion of the flesh. Juice therapists claim that the fruit fast
and vegetable juices can heal cases where the body is so
destroyed (for instance advanced tuberculosis, etc.) so as
to make absolute fasting difficult. Dieticians try to imitate the
chemical and liquid proportion in composition of fruit and
vegetables, in the artificial customary diet, but they can never
get the consumer to drink all the water to make the proportion right. They say you should drink at least eight glasses of
water a day, but who does? The human body has water as its
main element. Nature's sun-purified and sun-distilled water of
fruits, and vegetable juice is living water and the most needed
substance for replenishment in the living body. In nature the
water-is in living combination with the food, but the artificially
prepared dry foods (rice, bread, meat, potatoes, pastry, etc.)
are so strong that they burn out the digestive system rapidly. Fruits and herbs are naturally laxative, while this dry food
material will only make paste and glue clogging up the system
and start fermentation, putrefaction autointoxication, and make
the belly a cesspool of filth The study of autopsies shows that
most all people carry around 30, 40, or even more pounds of
morbid matter which is cemented to the walls of the intestines
preventing food assimilation. One starves more on the civilized diet, often, than the faster who periodically cleans out the
cemented mass so that food can be assimilated.


Publishers note: A strict juicy fruit diet is not recommended because it can cause severe tooth decay. A fruit diet
supplemented with vegetables, greens and cultured dairy
products like natural cheese and yogurt will prevent de-calcifi-
cation of the teeth and bones. The transition should be gradual
using cooked rice and potatoes, plus cooked vegetables. This
will allow the body to handle the excess toxic waste products
being eliminated. Foodless living is a special gift of God given
to very few people in religious history and is not to be emulat-
ed by others.

The carnivorous animals have a short alimentary canal; but man's is that of a fruitarian (in diet classification with the frugivorous monkey, ape, etc.) being some thirty feet long. The short alimentary canal of carnivorous animals gets rid of the carcass it eats very shortly, but man has the carcass, paste, and grease within him for days, if not cemented in for weeks, months or years till it is eliminated. Man wonders why he is sick!

Jesus, the Way, the Truth and the Life says, "Drink ye all of this, for this is my blood of the new testament which shall be shed for many unto remission of sins. And I say unto you, I will not drink henceforth of this fruit of the vine, until that day when I shall drink it new with you in the Kingdom of my Father." The "new" or fresh juice of fruits is to be shed and taken for remission of sins instead of the animal sacrifices of ancient and modern custom. Get your blood transfusion from the omnipresent Christ Life in the juice of fruits for that will give you life besides Life Everlasting.

After a few weeks of the juicy fruit diet one will notice the absence of passion, that is, one's thoughts are not attracted to sex, find little if any pleasure in it and, of course, there is a relief from the packing of the reproductive glands that continually breaks the reservoir of the fluid of life. After seven months without a loss of semen the vital fluid sac is sufficiently fortified and one can test for one's self the effect of different vegetable foods if one does not find the fruitarian regimen satisfactory. One should not use too many things at a time so that the experiments will be confused by foreign articles in combination. A few days constant use of any food will readily tell you if it is too rich, too stimulating or irritating by the relative over-secretion of the blood-builder fluid, stimulation of lustful thoughts and irritation of the urine if not of the food itself somewhere in the alimentary canal.

Jesus said: "For there are eunuchs who were born from their mother's womb: and there are eunuchs, who were made so by men and there are eunuchs who have made themselves eunuchs for the kingdom of heaven. He that will take let him take it." Though Jesus loved children and did not commit Himself about giving birth to them. He certainly sanctions the celibate life for the kingdom of heaven. Making oneself a spiritual eunuch, doing away with sexual passion through right living and sublimation of the sexual building force, is the object of Vitarianism. The Fountain of Youth is within you and as Jesus quotes the scriptures on believers, "Out of his belly shall flow rivers of living water." Reincarnationists would say: The eunuchs made by men are for sin or punishment of actions in past lives. In a sense this includes also eunuchs from the wasting of one's youth thru sexual abuse bringing on menopause and sterility. And there are the eunuchs born of their mother's womb, who have complete conservation without any difficulty, thru a gift.

A number of explorers into the wilds of South America found certain tribes of white Indians of unusual longevity, males of large physique and females free of menstruation. In a number of cases among primitive tribes of people which were of these remarkable characteristics in health, they lived on vegetable food only and were engaged always in physical labor. Also children brought up on vegetarian natural foods even in civilization in many cases do not have menstruation or seminal losses till the early twenties, if ever.

However, just not having passion and seminal losses is not the only thing to be desired and endeavored for. A ruinous life in sin will rapidly bring sterility and menopause. Vitarianism is a science to bring one back to the ecstatical feeling of living one has in pre-adolescent youth, and not the aching passion that will soon destroy one thru waste of substance in false pleasure. Also Vitarianism is not intended to be founded on scriptures of the dead. We have quoted scriptures realizing we live and teach in a dead artificial culture. The scriptures, alone, are dead. They have to be lived, to be true. Our teaching is for the Bible student as well as for those who feel, "The world is the best teacher, nature is the best book and God is the best friend," without ceremonies, authorities and holy personalities.

A modern physician states it without ecclesiastical language. "The act of generation is the beginning of death.

Throughout all forms of existence it is so. Many plants die as soon as the seed is mature. Man would surely die, once the seed became ripened and expelled, but man has the potentialities that are far greater than the insignificant plant. These potentialities have made man capable of producing millions of seeds before he dies. His task is not complete when he wastes one single seed. He has the capacity to go on, and in time the cells and tissues and nerves and the brain have degenerated so much because of a lack of replenishing material, that man dies. Our modern physiologists overlook the fact that one of the biggest causes of disease is the excessive indulgence in the sex act. The quantities of fluid lost by modern woman in their monthly flow is another subject that needs investigation. These fluids that are wasted have caused women to assume a minor role, lose her charm and become subject to many types of behavior completely foreign to man. She ages more rapidly. Strangely enough when she reaches the period of menopause, then she catches up and is able to outlive man. Each cell and each tiny organized body within the (human) form, requires a seed for its fertilization, and when the seed is unnecessarily discharged without, the form sacrifices the seeds required for more cells and more tissue."

In a subtropical climate vegetables grow all the year around. To perpetuate lettuce, cabbage, artichoke, chard, etc., we forbid it to go to seed by continually trimming off the seed buds and excess leaves. This makes the plant everlasting. If the plant is left to produce seeds it dries up and dies. The same is true of man. Fast and nip off the excess seed buds and flesh that wastes away one's regenerative substance.

LESSON V

GUIDE TO VITARIAN FOOD

The following chart is an attempt to give you a Guide to Vitarian Foods. This religious science has in view to discriminate spiritualizing, vitalizing, or Vitarian foods from degrading, devitalizing, demineralizing, stimulating or Passion-Producing foods. Vitarian foods generally have less than 2% protein, and more than 75% water. Water is our greatest food substance, and protein is the most unwanted substance, being the flesh producing element that devitalizes and degenerates the body. Mother's milk, a food intended by nature to nourish during the greatest need for growing material, has 1.60% protein and 87.75% water, and otherwise is a good guide to govern the requirements of the body. There are some exceptions, due to the high mineral content of some foods and other vitarian characteristics that one learns thru practice of the spiritualizing diet and we have indicated them on our chart.

Fruit is man's perfect food. It furnishes the greatest percentage of living water and the least amount of flesh-stimulating protein designed by the Creator for man's higher spiritual development. Living on the heavy passion-producing protein diet, man's thoughts are ever in the lower desires of the flesh. However, "the wisdom of the flesh is death but the wisdom of the spirit is life and peace." There is one exception shown in chart as protein, which is that of dried olives that are very alkaline and as a heavier food are very life-conserving. Other fruit mentioned when dried have a protein content exceeding 2%, but if soaked or used with juicy fruit give fine results. The fruit that is the downfall of fruitarians (which humorously we call the forbidden fruit of Eden) is the avocado. Because it is a fruit, fruitarians overdo it, not realizing it is used as a sex stimulant in South America. A small slice seemingly does no harm, but bit by bit a liking is developed for indulgence in irrational quantities. Foods marked VVV are 100%, Vitarian, good for fruit fasts of seven months, and general diet basis.

Herbs or vegetables are the next best food for man. They contain less living substance than fruit, and thus being less evolved, are harder to digest. This will be noticed in that on fruit juice, digesting in 2 or 3 hours, one sleeps only 2 or 3 hours. On a raw vegetable diet, requiring 6 hours to digest, one sleeps 6 hours. Fruit is for spiritual endeavors and vegetables for physical labor. One should adjust the diet to the kind of work one is doing. Most all herbs will be found to be vitarian. Chickweed, a common herb, found under trees is an example of a plant healing and vitalizing that can do much to remove seminal losses if picked before the seed forms.

| Food | Water | Protein | Vitarian | Passion Producing |
|------|-------|---------|----------|-------------------|
| FRUITS | | | | |
| Apples | 84% | 0.4% | VVV | |
| Apricots | 84% | 1.4% | VVV | |
| Avocados | 70% | 2.1% | | P |
| Bananas | 75% | 1.3% | V | |
| Blackberries | 86% | 1.3% | VV | |
| Cactus fruit | 79% | 1.4% | VV | |
| Cherries | 80% | 1.0% | VV | |
| Dates | 20% | 2.1% | V | P(?) |
| Figs | 79% | 1.5% | VV | |
| Grapes | 78% | 1.3% | VVV | |
| Grapefruit | 87% | 0.5% | VVV | |
| Huckleberries | 78% | 0.8% | VV | |
| Mangoes | 87% | 0.6% | VVV | |
| Pears | 84% | 0.6% | VV | |
| Plums | 79% | 1.0% | VVV | |
| Prunes | 81% | 0.8% | VVV | |
| Olives (dry) | 30% | 5.2% | VV | |
| Oranges | 87% | 0.8% | VVV | |
| Persimmons | 66% | 0.8% | VV | |
| Pineapple | 80% | 0.4% | VVV | |
| Raspberries | 86% | 1.0% | VVV | |
| Strawberries | 88% | 1.0% | VVV | |
| Tomatoes | 94% | 0.9% | VV | |
| Watermelons | 92% | 0.5% | VVV | |
| VEGETABLES | | | | |
| Artichokes | 79% | 1.8% | V | |
| Asparagus | 93% | 1.8% | V | |
| Beets | 88% | 1.2% | V | |
| Cabbage | 90% | 1.9% | V | |
| Carrots | 87% | 1.0% | VV | |
| Celery | 94% | 1.1% | VV | |
| Cucumber | 95% | 1.2% | VV | |
| Garlic | 64% | 6.8% | | P |
| Lettuce | 94% | 1.4% | VV | |
| Onions | 87% | 1.6% | | P |
| Potatoes | 75% | 2.1% | | P |
| Pumpkin | 90% | 1.1% | VV | |
| Swiss Chard | 92% | 1.5% | V | |

| Food | Water | Protein | Vitarian | Passion Producing |
|---|---|---|---|---|
| **MISCELLANEOUS** | | | | |
| Honey | 18% | 0.4% | V | |
| Sugar cane | 75% | 1.5% | VV | |
| Olive oil | | | V | |
| Vegetable oil | | | V | |
| Mushrooms | 89% | 2.6% | | P |
| Sorghum syrup | | | VV | |
| **CEREALS** | | | | |
| Barley | 14% | 11.1% | | PP |
| Corn, whole | 14% | 9.8% | | PP |
| Corn, green | 75% | 3.1% | | P |
| Corn, popped | 4% | 10.7% | | PP |
| Millet | 11% | 9.0% | | PP |
| Oatmeal | 7% | 16.0% | | PP |
| Rice | 13% | 7.8% | | PP |
| Rye, flour | 12% | 6.8% | | PP |
| Wheat, whole | 13% | 13.6% | | PP |
| Wheat, white | 12% | 10.2% | | PP |
| Bread, wheat | 35% | 8.9% | | PP |
| Wheat, germ | 12% | 35.7% | | PPP |
| Pumpernickel | 42% | 4.2% | | P |
| Sunflower seed | 7% | 14.2% | | PP |
| Sesame | 5% | 35.9% | | PP |
| **LEGUMES** | | | | |
| Beans, dried | 14% | 24.3% | | PP |
| Horsebeans | 14% | 18.0% | | PP |
| Garbanzos | 14% | 13.0% | | PP |
| Kidney beans | 15% | 22.8% | | PP |
| " (green) | 84% | 3.9% | | P |
| Lima beans | 10% | 18.1% | | PP |
| Peas, dried | 15% | 22.8% | | PP |
| Peas, green | 74% | 7.0% | | P |
| Soya beans | 10% | 34.0% | | PPP |
| String beans | 84% | 3.9% | | P |
| Almonds | 5% | 21.4% | | PP |
| Brazil nuts | 5% | 17.0% | | PP |
| Coconut | 14% | 5.7% | | P |
| Coconut milk | 92% | 0.4% | | VV |

| Food | Water | Protein | Vitarian | Passion Producing |
|------|-------|---------|----------|-------------------|
| **NUTS** | | | | |
| Filberts | 5% | 16.5% | | PP |
| Piñons | 3% | 14.6% | | PP |
| Walnuts | 2% | 18.4% | | PP |
| Peanuts | 7% | 29.8% | | PP |
| **ANIMAL PRODUCTS** | | | | |
| Cow's milk | 87% | 3.5% | | P |
| Butter | 11% | 1.0% | V | P |
| Cheese | 38% | 23.7% | | PP |
| Eggs | 73% | 12.5% | | PPP |
| Meat, average | 72% | 20.0% | | PPP |
| Chicken | 72% | 21.3% | | PPP |
| Fish, average | 80% | 18.3% | | PPP |
| Oysters | 86% | 6.2% | | PPP |

Sorghum syrup is a sweetener of a higher vibration and more pleasant taste than molasses and honey. Olive oil is best, though thru economic necessity coconut or vegetable oil may be more practical. True, in using corn, cottonseed, sunflower, etc., one destroys the seed, but these seeds should not be for producing human food as are herb and fruit seeds. Moreover, in extracting the oil the protein and the objectionable seed propensities are removed so as not to remain as a reproductive excitant. Butter, also having protein removed is not sex stimulating, though it is not Vitarian from the cow's viewpoint, and grazing land can be used more profitably in vegetable oil production or preferably in fruit culture. Grains and legumes should not be used. In case of necessity green (milk texture) corn can be used. Piñon nuts, hazelnuts, etc., in milk state seem tolerable moderately. Mature grains should not be eaten, but rather the sprouts of wheat, bean sprouts, etc. The sprouted seed becomes a living food, from its dormant state, turning the starch into digestible sugars and vitamins, besides dissolve the protein and seed propensity. The resulting vegetable, the sprouts of grains and legumes is of a texture similar to lettuce, etc. and instead of a few months necessary for a vegetable garden, a sprout culture takes only a few days. Even potatoes when mature may cause seminal losses, and yet immature new potatoes without full protein and starch texture may result neutral, acceptable as a cooked salad dressing. We do not recommend experimentation on these borderline foods, especially in the beginning when one is trying to remove seminal losses, and a habitual desire for these can only undermine the virtues of the ideal diet.

Years ago health commercialists sold us soya bean foods as a flesh substitute. Then they found no flesh substitute and only 2% protein necessary for hard labor. Then they developed the lecithin fad, "brain and nerve food", as an excuse to pacify the heavy protein desire. Sesame seed, with twice the protein content of beef, besides other specialties like popcorn, millet, etc., claimed to be alkaline, and tho not stimulating like meat, certainly are excess semen producing. The promoters of the mentioned foods we know personally to be well along in years and their claims of sex conservation thru such foods have deluded a number of young students. Foods that cause no losses in an older person, in youth of late teens, and in twenties can rapidly waste away the sexual vigor. Vitarianism is youth conservation not to be guided by veteran vegetarians raised on old heavy protein food and concepts, who are wasted away in substance tho they present their unsuccess to us as the truth.

Deeper analysis brings us to the conclusion that all stimulation of strength comes from the sexual force, which in turn gets it from the Solar energy in the air we breathe giving us our electrical dynamo in nerve force. The conventional food man eats, artificially stimulates the sexual center of force, that is, thru an excess of building material for the body, the reproductive animal instinct is awakened to use up the excess protein seed material, thru passion stimulating emotion which demands deep breathing that generates muscular energy to give the feeling of stimulated strength. However, instead of it giving a healthy body free from disease, this stimulation from food has only made man weaker and the more feebler in health. Modern civilized man, eating many times the food needed of a heavy protein concentration, including dry seed material, is least resistant to disease, weak, pot-bellied, toothless, and in physical degeneration, shameful to connect with the powerful healthy frugivorous ape.

## LESSON VI
## FEEDING FOR STRENGTH OR STIMULATION

The approach to the vital question of sex sublimation on which our health and spiritual development depends directly, has been sadly neglected, and faced with a negative denial in constructive avenues. Satan is able to intrigue more into sin thru man's rebellious hatred for secrecy. We do not cure a child from mischief by telling him what not to do, but rather thru positive intriguing suggestion in good actions. What interests people is why not to do something, rather than merely being told not to do it, and more can be done by constructive positive action rather than just destructive negation. We shall now frankly explain the how and why in spiritual action of the sex functions. Just as the lotus springs up out of slimy mud and blossoms into beauty, like the rose grows out of dung saturated earth to give forth wondrous fragrance, so the spirituality of man is reborn sublimated from the lower passionate and corruptible man.

First, we shall explain how stimulating foods weaken one, tho giving a false feeling of strength, and how with energy-generating and conserving foods one can generate health, strength, and spiritual power. Let us see what happens if we eat beef steak, or just any heavy protein such as beans, nuts, grains, etc. Immediately the body has a stimulating feeling of strength, we say the protein food gives us strength, so we exercise more and build up muscles and it is concluded that protein foods are thus necessary for health and strength.

Also, we notice that sexual thought or stimuli does the very same thing. A horse may be pulling a heavy load up the hill, becomes completely exhausted, and while otherwise unable to move on, the sight of a mare immediately gives the horse stimulation that enables it to go on in full strength. In school, we have noticed that the athletes with a beautiful physique are often those who are known as the well-sexed romantic type, in spite of what the coach says to them about dating out with girls during training. All know the exhilarating feeling that the presence or suggestion of the opposite sex gives, which often enables one to do what is otherwise impossible.

It is not that man is incapable of health and strength of apes and any other wild animal as there are continual reports of this being accomplished. The press of March 3, 1935 gave the report of a Joanna Mandrilla, who took to the wilds to become a "Female Tarzan" of super human strength. Several years after disappearing from her farm home in the Carpathian Mountains, she was captured with great difficulty, and found to refuse all food except flowers, plants, and grass. Again Aug. 28, 1946 it was reported that a 14 year old boy of the Syrian desert was found living on an exclusive diet of uncooked grass, roots, and water. He had a splendid physique capable of unbelievable feats such as running more than 40 miles an hour alongside a jeep. Besides these cases of uncivilized persons returning to the raw herb and fruit diet, in the United States there are many "raw fooders" and fruitarians, especially in California, who prove beyond a doubt that one cannot only live on a low protein herb and fruit diet, but also derive very remarkable cures, health, strength and spiritual benefits from it.

Right now in the United States, land of so much research in balanced diet, 90%, of the school children have dental decay. Investigations in the diet of Polynesians, known for fine teeth and physique, have shown that the substitution of grains for starchy roots and tubers that composed 85% of the calories formerly used, has resulted in decayed teeth in Hawaiian babies before they completely erupt. This shows that it is not the starch in food in general, but the protein and seed propensity accompanying the starch especially in grains, that make the difference in demineralizing the body. The studies of American Indians shows that those living on grains mostly have poor teeth, and the Zunis of the southwest U.S., whose native diet consisted of natural whole grain, mainly corn, with few vegetables and meat only occasionally are reported with dental caries in 75% of skulls examined. However, if the protein is without seed propensity, such as meat and fish, accompanied by eating the bones and cartilage, especially in raw state with all essential nutritive elements, there is not the rapid semen secretion in humans as is produced when seeds, especially milled grains, legumes, etc., are used. Only the absence of seeds accounts for good teeth in flesh eating races.

A dentist recommending preventive dentistry tells us that nuts have high potassium and phosphorous values, which tends to throw calcium out of the body increasing pyorrhea and dental decay. We notice that also where people chew up grains and nuts with teeth, they pass from the body without much assimilation, while the modern nut butters and milled grains not only do not exercise the teeth but are broken down to assimilate much of the protein, which wastes away the semen faster to give more disease on the rich digestible diet. Fruits with seeds in them like berries, tomatoes, etc., that are not removed in eating, do not give the effect of eating seeds because they pass from the body not assimilated as the seed remains intact and thus is propagated after being conveyed within animals to distant localities. Man creates an artificial, mechanical gizzard to grind his grains, nuts, seeds and suffers from too much fuel that burns up his system. Not eating the seed of plants and trees, is not only a theory on this being the forbidden fruit of Paradise, or philosophical idea on violating nature's intention for the seed, but as we have indicated, it is the latest scientific finding that research is stumbling on at last.

All this wasting away of teeth, hair, vital organs and reserve of energy to give the status of old age in the body is due to the stimulation one gets from protein and seed foods. One gets an oversupply of protein which draws minerals from the teeth, bones, and other tissues to manufacture the reproductive fluid, and thus the essential minerals are poured into the sewer thru sexual indulgency and seminal losses. The false feeling of stimulation of strength from protein-seed foods results in weakness felt after seminal losses or indulgence. As we have said carbohydrates are energy food as any dietician knows, and muscular power is produced by use of muscles, not eating food like the glutton, so that for health and strength it is essential to use plenty of energy-giving natural sugars and muscle-building exercise rather than the ordinary heavy diet. Notice the happy mental state and quick energy a child gets from eating sweets. The heavy grain and meat eating elderly person is only getting a stimulation like that of alcohol, tobacco, coffee, etc., giving a pickup for a moment, is continually wasting away the body in substance and disease.

We must begin to eat for strength, not for stimulation,-to give health rather than disease! Vitarianism is eating to give semen conservation which prevents body demineralization, conserving the teeth, eyes, hair bones, and body tissue from degeneration.

Our course has taken the basic method of semen conservation thru diet to prevent the unrestrained wasting away of the reproductive or renewing substance of our body. There are other methods of removing sexual lust that are not necessarily semen-conserving but do promote it in an indirect manner if used with the vitarian diet.

First is Mental Control, keeping the mind off of lustful thoughts. This method has been predominantly taught in the Christian celibate life along with the segregation of the sexes, and also is basic in Buddhist teachings. However, to remove passion that has an organic material cause by thought and mind is limited depending on a powerful mind capable of the seemingly miraculous. If the passions are controlled, the mental and material substance and energy has been wasted away through seminal losses, so little can be expected of the mind. One may hate and fight passion, only for it to gain and thrive pathologically wasting away brain and nerve substance, and paining the mind till the insanity drives them to brutal acts written about some religionist removing their organs, or the modernistic glandular surgical operations. Mind is a factor, but it is not the only approach and specific cure. Mental control of thoughts may prevent sexual indulgency, but this only gives rise to greater losses of semen through nocturnal emissions and menstruation.

Second, in the methods of semen conservation attempts is that of exercise. The ancient science of Yoga, established many millenniums ago, has established many forms of exercise to control any part of the body. These muscular contractions are called "Mudras". One of the most effective in results of an unusual nature being "Kechari Mudra" which is the practice of doubling the tongue backward till one stretches the tongue to be able to close the posterior nasal air passages so as to seal up one's existence enabling the Yogi to be buried for weeks at a time with no air, pierce his flesh without loss of blood and other remarkable performances. Other Mudras are chin contractions, abdominal muscular movements, enemas without mechanical aid, etc., all giving certain powers in physical dominion. The tongue contraction gives a higher mental current elevating thought, besides glandular and dieting control, but the specific way the Yoga achieves semen conservation is by an inner muscular contraction in the region of the semen containing sacs.

This exercise-is naturally done by everyone subconsciously, through fear of excitation at embarrassing occasions, and often religious mental control is achieved to the extent of frightening the sex muscles into control to prevent seminal losses. The Yogi on a light diet, consciously exercises the inner sex muscles just as one would exercise his arms, legs, chest, and back muscles by daily routine. By practice you will notice you can move the abdominal muscles, also you can contract the muscles of the anus at will and similarly the inner sex muscles are contracted so as to freely move the organs without touching them otherwise, in a manner similar to the heavy expanding throb of the heart or diaphragm, or just as one would raise the tongue in case of external erection. At first one may feel a slight upsetting feeling in the stomach, just as when one tries to wiggle one's ears or massage the abdomen through internal muscular contractions, but persistence little by little soon can give a dynamic control. At any time of sexual passion or erection this exercise can demonstrate fast results if persisted in till the inner sex muscles are tired, removing the nervous excitement besides build up the muscles so one can prevent loss at will under all conditions.

However, this exercise is definitely not a cure for eliminating sexual degeneration though one can remove menstruation, nocturation, nocturnal emissions and abusive indulgence with it. If the diet is such that it gives an overload of semen, and no outlet for it is given through ordinary sexual avenues, by such an exercise or surgical operation, the extra semen, principally albumin and protein decomposing into uric acid, fill the cell tissue of the body with waste and toxins, and overtakes the kidneys with diseases such as albuminuria, etc., with a constant loss of seminal substance in the urine. This muscular stoppage of passionate losses, or actual surgical stoppage if accompanied by the average diet, results in fatty flabby flesh characteristic of some celibates and eunuchs.

With an excessive tendency to kidney degeneration, the kidneys are not able to retain nutritive substances and the body loses its health-giving mineral salts in the urine.

Disease and Sin (Degeneration of body and soul) have one sure cure, the Fasting-Prayer taught by the Supreme Physician, Christ. The Baptism John taught was with water-cleansing in fasting and the harmonious omnilateral-therapeutic healing forces found in nature. Along with fasting, Faith-the desire to be healed rather than to sin-is the powerful healing force Jesus revealed in prayer to God. Besides the mental control and exercise, there are certain natural physical forces that should not be underestimated.

Physical labor uses up and thus eliminates excess semen in people who do heavy work if the amount of food is rationed, but if the work is allowed to only increase appetite and intake of food to an excess there is no greater mineral conservation.

Water, air, and sun baths are very neglected practices that have a very healing effect. The father of medicine, Hippocrates, equipped his sanatorium with a large solarium for heliotherapy to cure diseases. Benjamin Franklin, and many prominent people to our contemporary Winston Churchill have taken nude air baths every day. In South America uncivilized tribes of white Indians live on wild herbs and fruit, migrating according to the ripening of the fruit at different altitudes, are over 6 feet tall and often live to 200 years of age, and because they live completely nude, the women are free of menstruation; nor are there signs of sexual degeneration among these people. From olden times till the penetration of religion that taught people to associate sin with sex, the Finnish people have had the custom of "Sauna" steam baths, where men, women and children sweated and bathed together in winter, as they did in the summer in the hot sun and lakes completely nude. The Finns have been called the healthiest civilized race and certainly (except for drinking) it has no superior in morals in the western world, while the "evil flesh" hiding church people are known for their passionate life.

Sunlight destroys disease and passion. Science has shown that the greater the amount of sunbathing, the greater the amount of calcium and phosphorous is made available to assimilation from one's food, and naturists who spend most of their time with complete exposure of the body to the sun know that sunbathing reduces the food needed to one-half the amount needed when wearing clothes. The same is true in relation to passion, the wearing of clothes increasing the desire for sex, because covering up the body, so that it is bleached white just like lettuce, and other white leaved vegetables which makes them potent in the sex vitamin "E", creates the same reproductive propensity in humans. Moreover, the sight of the nude body is sanctifying, unlike the partially clad body, the ugly parts externally reminding us of shame in thoughts of sin just as the wounds on Christ Crucified refer us to thoughts of compassion He had for all.

Forsaking the fruitarian dietary plan God gave to man in Paradise, when he lived naked and unashamed, has given man's organized religion its continual status in sin and de-generation. In 394 AD the emperor of Greece ordered all the gymnasiums closed for the new prudish viewpoint toward the human body, and so thereafter the body temple of the Holy Spirit was veiled as unholy. And this made it more unholy as time went on from the immoral and unhealthy effects given by clothes. May Truth, which is holiness, conquer the world.

LESSON VII
VITARIANISM, THE FOUNDATION OF SPIRITUALITY

From the time of Hippocrates and the beginning of our era, to this day, medicine and religious doctrines have had their fads built on ever-changing human concepts adjusted to the tradition, custom, acceptability, and commercial value of the information they propagate. However, there are also the everlasting teachings of healing and redemption in our holy scriptures that will hold good for all times. Extracting all the teachings on healing our afflictions and conserving our health, we have a science of well-being which is most simple in prac-tice, but so difficult to preach or practice by either medical men or religious teachers.

Our western religion and medicine need to get at the root of sin. We have to crush the serpents head with the heel, or shall we say face the situation, not merely binding our eyes and hoping that by an "innocent" ignorance we may overcome sin. The naked truth will only make us free from sin. As we have been "harping away" continually in these lessons, it was the eating of the fruit-seed, that God forbids, which gave rise to passion and all the lusts that betake mankind. Partaking of fruit seeds, nuts, and vegetable seeds, grains, legumes, etc., besides eggs and of flesh itself, creates a super-abundance of flesh for one's body giving the desire to procreate profusely. Surfeiting, the overnourishing of the body which Jesus con-demns and is known as the cause of disease, causes the body to go to seed as its life seeks another perhaps health conserv-ing body to perpetuate itself in. Thus in the legendary Eden it is said that the original deathless man was cursed to always eating bread in sweat and sorrow, because of his violation that brought passion, shortening his life to 120 years, and finally man's action with women so displeased God, that He destroyed the sin-begotten civilization to the exception of Noah only. Think of all the sin in our world today, compared to that of Noah's day! It seems certain that our earth again awaits a cataclysmic "flood", or rather a fire, to cleanse it.

Now let us study the plan of redemption that the Lord Jesus Christ brought us as a gift of God to save man. The knowledge is nothing new, the regeneration of man being ancient wisdom. First He tells us to "Do Penance", meaning a sincere effort to pay or amend for our sins. As to what has to be accomplished He tells us: "Amen, unless man be born again of water and the Holy Spirit, he cannot enter the Kingdom of God. That which is born of flesh is flesh; and that which is born of Spirit is Spirit." The baptism with water is well explained by exemplification by Jesus as he went to John the Baptist and was bathed in the Essene ritual for commencement of his forty day fast for regeneration. The Second Birth requires a complete renewal baptizing with water all the cells of the body, besides the prayer-cleansing by Spirit. There is nothing that can spiritualize one into a new person more than abstinence taking fruit liquids or water alone along with meditation and contemplation of God in a pure natural surrounding. As we have often quoted, "Nothing shall be impossible for you ......thru fasting and prayer", that is, fasting and prayer achieve the omnipotence of the Heavenly King. We become Christ thru our second spiritual birth by going along with the Cosmic Law as did Jesus.

However, it is possible to heal to a certain extent "with words alone" as it would seem if there is grace of deep faith. Jesus would threaten an unclean spirit, "Deaf and dumb spirit, I command thee, go out of him, and enter not any more into him, etc." To some all this "Bible talk" may seem foolishness and laughable, but science is only discovering its truth today. Medical men now recognize that a great part of disease is only in the mind, that is, people become sick because of negative mental states. In other words they are in bad spirits, or rather bad spirits are in them, and they are unknowingly keeping themselves from being in the Good Spirit by their belief. The new healers again are casting out evil spirits as Jesus did, commanding these disincarnate entities that seek weak-willed bodies for expression to remove from the body that which they hold only thru a contagious fear, and with confidence in the healer, miraculously the body is healed physically with the establishment of the original owner in full control of his body. If you have tried every way for self-healing with no results, this very moment you may be healed by understanding that your battle with evil is due to disincarnate souls that, not having a body of their own to enjoy the worldly pleasures, seek your body to realize their desires. Knowing this to be the cause, pure holy thoughts and words can be used to send them away, besides fasting, which takes away the sensual foods they love; and thus is the most efficient weapon of dislodging evil spirits. Realize that it is these malicious spirits that give you the lower food desires for flesh, protein, and seed material, and the most difficult of all evils to overcome is the sexual lust because these disincarnates try every way to make one give them a body from your flesh thru sexual reproduction.

How do we know we are born of God, new and virgin in body, mind and soul, redeemed from sin? John Beloved Disciple of Christ tells us this very clearly,-"Whosoever is born of God committeth not sin; for his seed abideth in him, and he cannot sin, because he is born of God." This means that one is a Master of Life- or "Master Vitarian" having overcome seminal losses and passion in every way. The only true virgins are those who conserve their seed of internal regeneration. As Jesus stated it, "There are eunuchs who have made themselves eunuchs for the kingdom of heaven. He that can take, let him take it." The holy life is that of celibacy.

However, He also said, "Suffer the little children and forbid them not to come to me for the kingdom of heaven is for such",-showing that children are not the enemy, but should be loved by all. Rather, the purpose of the seed is for perpetuating youth within ourselves, instead of wasting it on pleasure and creating more short-lived creatures. Jesus tells us "death shall be no more" in his Kingdom, as did the prophets of old, meaning the short lives of people with a great number of births and deaths for the souls brought about because of sexual waste of substance, shall give way thru celibate regeneration, to a full life experience with hundreds of years of clear conscious knowledge to make them free for the ascension to God.

Only with mastery of life,--substance and energy conservation,-can we expect to realize that "They shall not hunger nor thirst" in our Heavenly Kingdom on earth. This is because

Christ tells us that those that enter the Kingdom of God, do so thru being born again, meaning that "Whosoever is born of God committeth not sin and the semen remaineth in him." This is scriptural proof and logic that when man is able to conserve his seminal substance he is born again to the highest spiritual plane in which there is no need of eating to replenish body substance that is destroyed in sex pleasure and disease.

The Life Abundant in which death comes no more is only possible through the cleansing baptism of water (fasting), and Spirit (prayer), that makes possible perpetual and complete semen conservation doing away with the necessity of food and other needs of mortals. Certain saints of the Catholic Church, Nicolas von Flue, St. Marian of Jesus, Theresa Neumann, etc., have proven this besides Yogis and Taoist masters who in cases have overcome the need of eating. As it is said, "there are bodies celestial and bodies terrestrial", that is, people who live an earthly life with mortal bonds in this life as well as those who become free sustained by Spirit living in a miraculous manner in privation of needs, heaven-wise.

Long ago Jesus warned us, "And as in the days of Noah, so shall also the coming of the son of man be. For as in the days before the flood, they were eating, drinking, marrying, and giving in marriage and the flood came and destroyed them all." Has there ever been a greater need for saints that live the holy life of celibacy and fasting than at present? The majority are content in just believing in Jesus as a true story, but will not do any of the things he claimed necessary to be His disciple or to receive the glory of His kingdom. Basically Christ's Gospel is on dieting and the celibate life, which he continually emphasizes in the scriptures. It is easy to see something else, little points that need very little sacrifice to follow to be a so-called Christian.

As we have in Romans VII, which in this case is easier to understand in the King James version, "For to be carnally minded is death, but to be spiritually minded is life and peace."

Not only is what we call "Vitarianism" the doctrine of Christ, who is the Life, or "Vita" of the world as taught by Jesus, but many centuries before the Yogis had long taught it under the name "Brahmacharya" or celibate purity. They teach that wasting of the semen brings death, that the semen is the real vitality of man, that through conservation one can live as long as one desires, that absolute control over the sex force gives all powers in miracles, and Brahmacharya (freedom from sexual thoughts or desires) is the foundation for Spirituality and God Realization. Yogis practice (1) Deep breathing to get a super-abundance of cosmic energy "Prana", (2) Celibacy to conserve it, and (3) Meditation to sublimate it, raising up the "serpent" energy to give them God-Vision, Divine Ecstasy, and other spiritual powers. The lower sexual force is transmuted into spiritual force. Not only is Brahmacharya claimed to be the best of penances, but also the supreme of medicines by the Hindus.

Buddhism, the philosophy with the most followers, also regards Brahmacharya as a basic teaching. Gautama Buddha said that lust is the cause of all sentient beings, that is the basis of temporal things, including what we call nature. Nature is the product of lust, evolution, the battle of passionate desires. "All who are born must die." "The origin of suffering is lust, passion, and the thirst for experience that yearns for pleasure, that leads to continual rebirths. The Liberation from desire, the deliverance from passion is the annihilation of suffering." All creation has come into existence thru lust, said Buddha, and now in Vitarianism we teach how to annihilate lust and passion by feeding the body but at the same time starving out passion. "Destroy birth, and death and old age will cease", the Light of Asia would say cautioning against motives in thought or action involving sex.

The Buddha, giving instruction to the disciples says, "Raw grains and meat he does not accept", along with exhorting abstinence from sexual lusts, which is like other sages (Pythagoras prohibiting disciples to eat beans, etc.) have warned the disciples of the common sex stimulating foods. Raw grains and nuts have more nourishment and seed propensity than cooked grains and nuts, but in all cases the elimination of these forms of seed gives the complete key for doing away with passion besides seminal losses.

We read of certain Taoist masters living without eating for 2 or 3 years by living celibately with young virgins. Living without losing any of their seed which is caused by the common disease of over-nourishment, they do not need to replenish their substance by eating food to build semen and blood. It is seen that the sexes living together with chaste endeavor, create a magnetic interchange of sublimating emanations, but in some cases the separation of the sexes in asceticism has led to hidden ambitions resulting in hidden actions, and the separate polarities being so concentrated, result in sterile higher motives in the opposite polarity.

Carnal union of the sexes is sin, and if an individual is so dominated by animal instinct that he has to be segregated like male and female animals, he is not ready for the spiritual life. However, it is the blending of the higher qualities that creates spiritual perfection. Gal. III:28 "There is neither male nor female. For you are all ONE in Christ." The carnal union of the sexes creates the accelerated aging and degeneration, noticeable immediately after marriage of a few years, while this could be avoided by continuing love on a spiritual plane which can actually youthify those involved, by the sublimation of the conserved vitality and substance within themselves. Ecstatic rapture is also necessary for existence without food. A love rapture may wear off in 2 or 3 years in the temporal spiritual union of souls limiting the time of food abstinence, as we refer to the Taoists example. However, the Divine Ecstasy of love and gratitude extended to all persons and things instead of one person, gives an exotic realization of God as Life Essence everywhere present. There is nothing more blissful than to be ecstatically in Love with God! This supreme Joy is Omnipotent, because it begins with, the loss of appetite (Fasting) and adoration, (Prayer) experienced by worldly lovers also. "Nothing will be impossible for you by fasting and prayer."

LESSON VIII

MAN'S REAL FOOD

That fruit is man's perfect and only real food, we have explained from spiritual and scriptural authority in some of the preceding lessons, but it is not something only understood by legends about a Garden of Eden. Due to cataclysmic climatic conditions brought upon man (proven by remains of tropical trees and vegetation found buried even in the arctic zone) man has found it necessary to choose substitutes for fruit where it is not planted. However through adaptation to the inferior foods such as flesh, grain, eggs, milk, etc., they have become the habitual diet, so that they seem to be the only satisfying foods. But just as suffering is allotted out to some souls placing them into hostile climates of ice and snow with no vegetables, not to speak of fruits, so also some individuals do not harmonize with the ideal diet, because they only have earned to deserve the suffering that results from being fed by disease-producing foods. Thus they would perhaps only suffer on the ideal fruit diet if they were forced to it, with no better results than on the disease-producing diet, because of psychological degeneration from a negative mind. But let us seek perfection and not the old sad state of the world.

So instead of the legendary basis for the dietary foundation of man, let us look at it biologically, physiologically, ethically, if not esthetically, to determine if man was not frugivorous in the beginning as well as now.

Man is not a Flesh Eater or CARNIVOROUS because the molar teeth are not pointed for tearing flesh, the saliva is not acid for meat digestion, the intestinal canal needs to be four times shorter to prevent rapid putrefication of the carcass eaten and in many respects man is not physiologically capable of meat-eating habits for health. Not only is the sight of flesh devouring naturally repulsive esthetically to humans, but its persistence will cause a hardening of the heart psychologically so as to promote cruelty increasingly till even the killing and torture of human beings becomes a liking of the animal carcass eater. Putrefication begins immediately after the animal is killed, and everyone knows the offensive stench of the dead animal carcasses besides that of the excrement of carnivorous animals which our senses should warn us against carnivorism. However, the urine in animal tissues, though known for its poisonous nature, is craved by the meat-eater (as alcohol is by alcoholics) making bouillon cubes (chemically urea) good to stimulate appetite in medical patients. As to medical findings for the nutritional value of meat, it may have a very recommendable chemistry, but so does dung. In South America where sanitary facilities are not available most often the dogs scavenge the streets and most probably they get enough protein and other dietary necessities just as well as on a meat diet to keep them alive, though both are second hand foods. We are not trying to be offensive to anyone but hope to illustrate a fruitarian viewpoint in answer to whether one does not get hungry for beefsteak or a hamburger on vegetable foods. There is no substitute for fruit.

Man is not perfectly destined to consume animal products. A great many have the idea that to be a vegetarian is to live on eggs and dairy products. To keep animals for slaughter is unquestionably inhumane, but to keep chickens overfed to produce a continual unnatural forcing of eggs and to have a cow as a perpetual wet nurse for man, to some may not seem cruel to animals. However, let me present a view similar to that of temperance people who say that light drinks like beer and wine are worse than hard liquor like whiskey, because the beer and wine is easy to begin with developing a taste for the strong drink which is repulsive to commence with. Similarly milk and eggs, though with seeming innocence as to cruelty, keep the "vegetarian" a slave to desire for animal foods, while the complete abstention from animal products breaks one from the animal natured association of pleasantness to the odor of gravy, lard frying, besides actual cooked carcass. To nullify their argument, animals could be raised without life-long slavery to being cooped in wire cages for egg giving, being milked and herded around every day, etc. by letting them multiply naturally on the open cattle range as the Indians did the buffalo, and having them killed painlessly rather than the objectionable cruel slaughterhouse practices. But this is only to point out the logic that whether painlessly or painfully obtained, animal products are not the food for man. Have mercy on all creatures including the chicken and cow by not making their suffering on earth necessary because of man's appetites.

Now what is the difference if we eat a chicken's leg, breast or its embryo innocently called an egg? In all cases the chicken raising results in the slaughter of the chicken in the end and the egg consumer patronizes this. We have the smart retort from the clever "vegetarian" that they only eat unfertilized eggs, not destroying life and one of the shocking reports is that a certain leading "fruitarian" advocates the fruit of a "Cackle-fruit!" All we have to say is, unfertilized eggs may not be directly as guilty of bird abortion, but thus it is eating the tumorous growth or cyst of a chicken. An egg has the same putrid smell as other forms of rotting flesh and worse if it is only a chicken's tumor. Though eggs, along with flesh, fish and fowl are acid-forming putrefying foods that many medical doctors admit are a great cause of so much of our common diseases, milk is often classified by these as a perfect food. However, what is milk, but a modified cow's blood secreted for the sustenance of its young. At least the mammary modification of the cow's blood was intended as a food for something, not being so toxic as flesh so brutally procured, but how unfortunate that man the superior animal suckles himself and his young from the lowly cow or goat. Certainly it is not esthetically natural to find human beings nourishing from a cow's teats, especially when well able to find food for themselves!

We are very much in accord to Vegetarianism. Carnal food produces carnal desire, resulting a carnal mankind and its pitiful carnage. But vegetarianism is not the complete solution to the world's evil passions.

Witness India and other vegetarian populations very laudable for their pacifism, yet are spoken as being in need of birth-control. They live on grains mainly. Seed eating produces high seed propensity, reproductive or carnal desires also.

As we have told you before, man is not a GRANIV-OROUS animal because he does not have a gizzard, but is supposed to chew his food with the teeth which are not adapted by milling of grains. Nor does it help if man is so ingenious as to invent ways to mill the grains and other seeds and heat them to make them palatable, as this gummy soft paste is the same thing as used to stick wall paper and it certainly constipates or sticks on the intestinal walls. Besides clogging up the intestinal tract and filling the system with mucous, grains saturate the organism with calcareous deposits. Dr. T. de la Torre says, "According to Doctors Densmore, Robotam, De Lacy, Evans, Bubler and others, grain foods, especially cereals contain large amounts of earthy matter in the form of carbonates and phosphates of lime and magnesia which, when eaten abundantly, are very detrimental to health and shorten life. They are the prolific causes of digestive disturbances, hardening of the arteries, gout, and rheumatic affections and premature old age." And the taste of grains in natural state is similar to crude earth so is it any wonder that they fill one with the heavy earthy material deficient of the soft elastic body tissue substance, though this brittle inorganic substance does serve well for the building of the abundant feather and bone growth of birds.

By now some will say, I am trying to indicate that man should live on grass. No, I would not say man is HERBIVOROUS, though living on herbs is the easiest and least harmful substitute for a fruit diet. The roots, the stem and somewhat the leaves contain the sap or blood of the plant carrying earthy matter from the earth to the leaves to be made organic thru the work of the sunlight, so they are not completely as pure a food as fruit which stores the perfected organic food to tempt the transportation of the seed in the fruit without harm to the original plant. We do not claim that ordinary grass can be eaten as it is; like the horse does,-because the fibers are too tough for man's digestive system, but man has cultivated a great variety of soft succulent herbs we call vegetables besides using fire to prepare the tougher ones, so as to be able to adapt to any part of the earth where vegetation can be found. We have experimented ourselves, besides the findings of Christian saints and Tibetan yogis, on living on wild herbs such as nettles, dandelions, chickweed, watercress, sour dock, etc., that is edible greens found anywhere on earth that produces vegetation to find that there is no reason to say we cannot live on the herb and fruits diet because fruit is not found everywhere. Most people do not deserve luscious fruits and should do penance by the less pleasant diet of herbs for the dietary sins committed in the past, or scientifically spoken, mineralize their bodies and get back the natural sense of taste.

Fruitarianism is a self-evident fact. Casting aside all our acquired appetites let us see what has nature prepared as a perfect food. Certainly man has no real desire for raw flesh of animal carcasses; the raw egg rather than a food is used to create vomit; man should live independent of animals, nor should he destroy sentient life; grains and seeds are not naturally edible and cause diseases; and vegetables though more healthful than others, have to be combined in salads, cooked, etc., to be liked, while the fruit of the tree is ready to serve, delicious without further preparation and naturally health-giving. All other things have other purposes, but fruit alone has one purpose only, destined only for food to whoever can be tempted to partake and thus scatter the seed. However, the hasty deduction that some fruitarians take, in saying that the fruit of the tree is even the seed, bark and leaves, has led many to bad results. If anything from a tree were fruit, then nuts, coffee and cocoa beans, cinnamon, quinine tea leaves, etc., are also the intended food "fruit" for man's diet. As it is, nature put toxic substances in the other parts of the tree to protect the tree, while the fruit was selected for the greatest purity. The fruit has the sole purpose of attracting living beings to carry off the seed by partaking of the fruit, while the leaves and bark are parts of the tree which injure or destroy the tree if taken away, and the seed or nut is for the propagation of the tree though it does serve as food for the lower fast propagating short-lived mice, squirrels, birds, etc.

Man is supposed to be a "thinking animal", but if he thought about it, he would not start so commendingly on his big breakfast each morning with chicken embryo, pig's buttocks, cow blood secretion and plant seeds (eggs, ham, milk, and cereals) whose thought is even vomit provoking contemplating the animal carcass that it represents. Now we have compared man with lower animals to show he is not carnivorous, etc., yet we do not classify men by the ape saying he should eat what the ape does. By putting man to the ape way of living would be turning to the devolution of man instead of the regeneration of man. Man is not a superior ape, but the ape came from the degeneration of the original perfect man created by God, and this degeneration came from eating nuts, and other forms of seeds and protein that build flesh and sensuality at the expense of the brain. Man is much more delicately built and of a finer sensitive nature unlike the brute hairy ape, and because of this finer nature his food should be devoid of the elements that build the grosser nature found even in the frugivorous apes who include nuts, etc., in their jungle diet besides fruit, the perfected food.

Because of the habitual belief indoctrinated into contemporary diet students, they bring up protest, saying that taking nuts from the fruit diet would take away its source of protein. Science tells us that every living cell contains protein so really there is no food that does not have some protein. The point we are trying to bring out is pertaining to the amount and quality of the protein. We wish to again quote the words of a leading naturopathic writer: "The minimum protein requirement varies according to the vitality of the body cells and the kind of food one is eating. When the body is in a high state of purification and preservation and one lives mostly on vital foods, the disintegration (death) of the body cells is much slower than when the body is in a diseased condition and the food consists mostly of dead cells from animal bodies and altered by the excessive heat during the cooking process. On the other hand, when we eat natural foods which has not been submitted to the destructive cooking process, its cells are vital and capable of reconstructing the disintegrated tissue much more rapidly and efficiently and with a much smaller quantity of food. I have repeatedly observed in myself and in others that when the body is in a high state of purification as for instance after fasting or a purification diet, one increases weight rapidly on one-half the amount which physiologists consider to be the minimum protein requirement. On the other hand persons whose cellular tissues are in a high state of morbidity and decay disintegrate very rapidly and need a larger amount of food to replace the rapidly dying cells of their body. "I have learned to tell the state of decay of a certain person's body by finding out the amount of protein he needs to maintain his normal weight." Dr. T. de la Torre is right this far but when he turns around later to contradict this and insist that one cannot live on either fruit or vegetables alone because they do not have enough protein, we wish to give correction.

We do not say that one should try to live on a few ounces of fruit at each meal or the same accustomed volume as is needed on the heavy concentrated food. A coolie with a bird-sized stomach can live on a small handful of rice or beans, but our alimentary system is much larger, capable of expansion also through use. Gradually the omnivorous anatomy grows into becoming frugivorous, and the advantage in health is fast seen because of the greater intake of living water that cleanses the cells as the food nourishes. On heavy concentrated food you feed continually, but the waste piles up over-working the eliminating system till finally there is a breakdown to give various diseases. Fruit has the necessary cleansing agents to match the amount and quality of its protein.

LESSON IX

DEGENERATE FOOD, DEGENERATE BODY, DEGENERATE MIND

God created the perfectly evolved food, fruit, thru an evolutionary process that refines and sublimates the grosser substance from the earth to become the perfect tree ripened fruit that can be digested in two or three hours. But alas, so imperfect himself, man seeks not the perfected things, but goes to the inferior immature and grosser things in life and in eating. Rather than being perfect as the Father intended, he insists on living imperfectly and blames his suffering and sorrow on God's "wrath". Rather than the perfected, predigested fruit, he seeks to get the tree's nourishment in the green leaves, seeds, roots, fungus, and that, most often secondhand after being used by animals, thus eating their milk, eggs, and flesh. He has never stopped to think that this requires two or three times the time for digestion of pure food besides needing many times more energy than fruit to assimilate. So you see for the sensual pleasure gained from passionate foods, man's body energy supply, thinking power, mental happiness, and time for spiritual life are all lost in his physical activity of work to obtain this really expensive, troublesome and enervating diet.

Using the lower parts of plants the digestive system has to evolve the substance into the assimilable food that fruit already is, just as leaves, stem and roots do in the plant to perfect the fruit. Taking away the interior physical labor in man caused by the inferior diet, there is more freedom and power for the spiritual life. Experience tells me, the Higher Life is promoted by higher food, that is, foods that are spiritually conducive make the spiritual life practical and essential.

However, the grosser foods seem essential to mortal man. As we explained in Lesson VI, man likes the heavy protein diet because it stimulates a passionate feeling of strength by an abundance of reproductive fluid, just as sexual losses produce weakness. Eating the grosser foods (meat, seeds, etc.) man enjoys the stimulation for sexual lust, shedding blood, and other lower passions. From that we see the reverse statement true also, that is, to enjoy sexual lust, bloody fighting, and other lower passions, he needs grosser foods such as meat, seeds, etc.

Now, what we are trying to explain is that if man were on the path of spiritual perfection, he would only choose the perfect foods for him, but rather he chooses and is very much attached to the passion producing foods. That lower passion requires the lower passion-producing food is seen first in that to fortify sexual indulgence people eat eggs, steaks, etc., to replace the protein and mineral substance thus destroyed by the loss of the semen. In any kind of criminal, emotions that create worry in the conscience causes the organism to labor destroying brain cells that are irreplaceable besides nerve and other body tissue, so from this it can be seen that even theft and deception eat away one's organism fast, making this lower type of man require more of the grosser seed and protein foods. Finally may we say, that to participate in bloody fighting, and in a lesser degree, anger and work of extra exertion, one requires protein to replace the body cells injured in the fighting, besides nerve and body cells lost by anger and exertion beyond tolerance. Not only is it logical that animals who kill should live on their slaughter, but the slaughtered flesh enables them to rebuild their own flesh where they were injured. From this we see that man is to get away from using foods that accommodate his life as a killer, if he is to get away from killing itself. To get away from lower passions of any kind, he has to get away from the passion-producing diet that naturally inhibits the purer life.

The new "scientific finding" on the radio and papers about reducing is advertised as a high protein diet treatment. They claim excess of protein in the diet literally burns up excess fatty tissue! People will do anything to lose "ugly unsightly fat". What happens when the person takes on extra protein and other semen, blood and body building substances is that nature demineralizes the body faster thru sexual losses and abuse, and one becomes thin and dried up just as the lewd do thru much abuse. Just as the priests and other people living in continence, the ordinary person who does not have an extra sexual life or uses the extra protein of the ordinary diet to endure extra heavy labor, this extra nourishment is stored on the body for future use. But now "science" has a way to produce unconscious seminal losses, rather than openly advocate sexual indulgence and other ways to destroy one's substance. They promote the idea that only the unsightly fatty tissue is burned up leaving only good solid flesh, yet how about the findings that excess protein in the body converts into uric acid and other poisons, which means the fatty tissue degenerates from diseased conditions into a lesser size or volume. Rather than putting the extra weight to use in exercise, they say that that would not reduce but further fatten one by causing one to eat more. So again by giving another kind of a disease we destroy symptoms of the first kind of disease, but later after having wasted away the body because it became too fleshy, they wonder why they become sterile at 40. One may abuse the body so as to need an abundance of protein for normal weight, and vice versa, use extra protein to abuse the body to keep it from overweight, but one cannot get good solid weight only from eating only protein foods.

In the last lesson we began to show that the state of

decay of a person's body can be determined by his need of protein for normal weight. Now we have shown that also moral degeneration determines the amount of protein and other lower foods a man craves and actually needs to keep up the evil life. The fire of passion only burns when it is fed. The fighters become more blood thirsty if fed meat. Immoral foods favor an immoral life.

However, we observe also that not only does degeneration of the body cells come from disease caused by abuse of physiological laws, or from abuse of moral laws, but any tearing down of the body cells such as experienced in extra heavy labor creates a craving for reproductive substance to replace the used up body tissue. Man toils with sweat on his forehead because he has deserted the garden with every fruit and lives on the lower foods of hard labor such as grains for bread, meat from killing, etc. And that it is a fact that it is the conservation of the reproductive substance that builds the blood from the heavy diet of grains, meat, etc., can be seen in the fact that when the participants exert themselves to the utmost physically and often mentally, the reproductive fluid is used up entirely in the body without uncontrollable passion or even desire to destroy more of it sexually. However, in this we are not giving an argument against doing labor because it uses up the sexual substance, as the reproductive fluid was originally intended for reproducing our own body anew continually or eternally, though not with such drastic changes as created by 16 or 18 hours of heavy mental or physical exertion. In fact we know that vegetarians suffer less from bodily injuries and have more endurance than meat eaters, indicating that the more purified organism can do better without much protein in the long run, though needed. The original state of man free of sin, to be called Paradise or Heaven, does not require man to make exertions in fighting and nursing wounds from killing, replacing lost seminal substance, worrying or enacting retribution in stealing or deceiving, and working at heavy labor from sunrise to sunset to keep up this vicious cycle so as to have the heavy diet that produces these passions. The Celestial Man is a man with the Superior Mind (one with the Supreme Mind), not laboring in confusion physically and mentally, as is mortal man in his delusion ever enervated by his useless efforts against the will of his Creator.

Study the statements we have pointed out as being true as they are and how they are also true vice versa. We maintain that the State of the mind is the state of the body and also the state of the body determines the state of the mind, because the two are essentially one. Perfect the mind and the body is perfected noticeably; perfect the body and the mental outlook is rosy also; and yet it is the perfection of both that means perfection beyond the old status into rebirth of new mind and body. Mediocre ideals, half status conceptions of only mind or body, needed for perfection, give only mediocre, half status results.

BLOOD "Don't delay, give some blood today!" How blood thirsty can our civilization get? "Give to a Yank who gave" If they must resort to actual cannibalism, why could they not consume the blood they shed of their victims in killing, satisfying their blood thirst right there in the battlefield instead of ruining our day with continual pleas for blood. But the sad thing about it is that some gladly give their blood to these professional killers rather than give food to the innocent but starving in Asia while we are living in luxury and abundance. Save the innocent, not the blood-stainedness.

LESSON X

VITARIAN MENUS

"But Johnny, what do you eat! You say you don't use any kind of animal food, not even milk and eggs, and then no nuts, nor grains meaning no bread, etc., eliminating all the foods we have to use on a diet!" This is more or less like what some exclaim after a hurried glance at our diet system. Though there are hundreds of varieties of vegetables and fruits, they do not appear to be food for the diet in the dena- tured sense of taste of civilized man. How far man has erred from his original diet obtained by eating his fill from only one tree in a meal.

"But what do you eat ?" Yes, I will be so romantic, so

mystifying, and so seemingly fictitious as to relate that in the summer when fruit is abundant, I make a complete meal out of only one kind of fruit, and eat fruit for months on end with no other food. Though I have scarcely gone 3 years on fruit alone, this I have only interrupted because good fruit is seasonal in availability. One meal can be a large fruit bowl of fresh peaches, apricots, apples, grapes, watermelon, or other fruit that is of an agreeable balance in taste to eat alone.

"But don't you ever drink water? Don't you ever get thirsty?" people ask me in their gifted imagination of my sufferings at abstinence! Thirsty!-when the reason we favor fruit is for the 80% to over 90% content of nature's purest distilled water. For good health we are told to drink 8 to 10 glasses of water besides water in soup, milk, etc. But it is in the fruit that we get this needed extra water naturally in the purest cell-cleansing properties.

And with my confession of so diluted a sustenance, they ask me with a feeling of satisfaction of thinking they have sprung an intellectual trap, "Where do you get energy and strength?" Energy?-when fruit is a natural source of pure sweet sugar the instant energy giver. As to strength, that is a question of use rather than food proven by the fact that the heaviest eaters are the weakest and most diseased. An athlete depends on exercise for building and maintenance.

Finally feeling there is some disillusion to be found still to all this, they inquire, "How do you keep your weight up? On fruit alone we would lose weight." Would they? This reminds me of an instance when I told someone of my weight being nearly 200 pounds and they answered that among other reasons for this I was abnormal. To have been 200 pounds in their case or for average person would have been abnormal but for my height, 6' 4", I was not abnormally overweight as they imagined, nor was I underweight as medical standards would indicate for my height. Let me assure you that the fruit diet is one of the best ways to acquire plump cheeks; flesh on your bones and it is not at all a reducing diet as some have falsely imagined, though it will purge unnecessary weight in body toxins from one's person. For each food there is needed a special chemical secretion for digesting it. This is why one should eat one food at a time, favoring thorough digestion of it by a specific digestive juice.

But with the conglomeration of dozens of foods of even deadly compositions; how are the digestive juices to be made suitable for the digestion of all the varieties of foods. Our man has become a processing plant for garbage disposal. If the many course dinner of the wealthy were mixed together, steak, ice cream, wine, pastry, etc., would it not only be fit as garbage, and is that not what is done in modern civilized man's stomach? Simplicity in diet is one of the most important health rules.

In spite of the ideals of one food at a time we try to avoid monotony by various combinations that are not only primarily simple but harmonious in satisfying genuine hunger. Certain foods mix well and seem to need one another at times for liking. After our fruit meals let us mention the following Vitarian meals.

I.      Strawberries with cream made from bananas.

2.      Tart varieties of apples diced with soaked raisins.

3.      Raisins with carrots.

4.      Dried olives with raisins, dates or figs. Also use olives in salads.

5.      Tomatoes with cucumbers, besides with all salad vegetables are fine.

6.      Salad oil, preferably olive oil, is to be used with all salad vegetables.

7.      Grated carrots with either cabbage, lettuce, celery or cauliflower as a salad mixed with oil, lemon or tomato juice, and sweet fruit dessert.

8.      Any white leaved vegetable such as cabbage, let-

tuce, etc., with tomato juice, salad oil, etc., eaten with cooked squash or pumpkin.

9.      Grated carrots, leafy salad vegetables in salad eaten with cooked greens, artichokes, and other less starchy vegetables.

All salads are raw unless mentioning cooked articles and though the live food diet is recommended always, summer especially, in winter we have found it sometimes preferable to use cooked vegetables with the raw salads sparingly. Vegetables that may be cooked are greens of all kinds, the outside leaves of cabbage and cauliflower, chard, artichokes, squash, pumpkin, etc., which would not be utilized anyway if not prepared by cooking, and in the case of the greens being acclaimed most nutritious in the parts not ordinarily used. However, these cooked vegetables should be used as a raw salad dressing, and not indulged in as the main dish, which should be 80% raw or living food. When one is changing to or from the 100% fruit diet of summertime, before using the cooked vegetables that contain a light starch as the main carbohydrate, one can make all raw salads with honey or sorghum syrup, etc., in them. I have been criticized for using honey with cabbage when the means of subsistence got low, (sorghum and lettuce would have been better) but I have found such a balance of minerals with carbohydrates satisfactory for energy and building minerals.

Had we used the salad with peanuts, nuts or whole grains (customary of vegetarians) the result would have favored the contemporary dietetic ideas but thus giving pathological seminal losses that orthodox dieticians do not pay any attention to. Also the natural sugar and salad combination is better for preventing intestinal packing which soft cooked semi-starchy vegetables even favor. This is why potatoes, sweet potatoes, etc., though not rapid in influence, are not satisfactory for a constant diet. As to onions and garlic, some say since one needs so little they should be harmless, yet we have found them a raw foodist's drug, creating a foul odor in the user in spite of the good claimed for them. In the east Yogis classify garlic, onions, and other sharp flavored herbs as passion producing foods.

The average vegetarian complains that they have trouble finding food while traveling. We have found the very opposite true, if the mind is well controlled. Living in rural places, away from the centers of travel, one does not usually find foods ready to eat for vegetarians. However, when traveling one can always find dried fruits if not fresh ones. Any grocery has raisins and if one looks ahead he can carry a few packages of figs, dates, etc., besides apples, etc., which would cause no embarrassment as would trying to eat a strange salad on an airliner or bus.

Not only do we recommend some near "natural" (honey, sorghum syrup, etc.) sugar with salads, but also in drinks. The true product is an orange, though often we will try to make an artificial orange juice with natural sugar and water, with lemons, green oranges, etc. However, in spite of the substitute for the most natural, one finds these honey-lemon-ades, orange-ades, etc., alone substantial for holding one up with a cleansing regimen for weeks at a time. The same is true of the herb teas such as made with mint leaves, chamomile, etc. The hot water overcomes the mental illusory appetite by relaxing and soothing the internal digestive organs. Some vegetarians pretend to practice moderation with starches, but when feeling low and depressed, like the drunk keeping the bottle around, they go on a "spree" consuming bread by the loaf, nut butter by the jar, etc. What they should have done was had their cupboard supplied with herbs and sorghum syrup and there would have been beneficial results instead of the contrary. Some raw foodists claim it a problem that in winter they are tempted to cook foods, having to warm by a fire any way, but the cooking temptation can be profitably consumed in using herb teas rather than going all the way to tortillas, baked potatoes and beans.

It is sad that our commercial system has given us green fruit on our markets, and only ripe seed and grains for food manufacture. It should be the other way around, ripe fruit only and non-ripened grains and seeds for food manufacture if any. Only ripe fruit is perfectly digestible with its concentrated fruit sugar, and the same is true of immature vegetable foods like sorghum and sugarcane, germinated seeds used for making malt syrup, excluding the ripe seed of any kind. The only usable element of the ripe seed we have had any satisfactory results from is the oil.

Once one becomes adjusted to a natural diet of one kind of fruit at a meal, for instance figs, grapes, apples, etc., one will be able to rely on the same natural foods in simple combinations to supply the body's needs in minerals and vitamins. One does not need to be a graduate dietician to select mineralized and vitaminized foods once the natural intelligence of taste is restored.

LESSON XI

WHY REGULATE DIET TO CONSERVE SEMEN

The object of the Vitarian Diet can be briefly defined as conservation of the seed of life, or the seminal (reproductive) fluid of the body. But why conserve the human seed? Though, with the help of some young colleagues, we are establishing a tangible science on how to eat to contain one's strength and life force, perhaps we have not explained thoroughly the purpose of human seed conservation.

If one should ask a well-educated medical doctor or an illiterate hillbilly the purpose of the human seminal fluid, the answer would be the same, that is, they would say it was only for reproduction. They observe the animals of the laboratory and of the barnyard and conclude that human reproductive power is identical in purpose to that of animals. However, a few scientists have observed that only civilized man and domesticated animals are easily excited sexually, the opposite being true of wild animals in their natural state, and man's reproductive instinct is aroused at all times rather than seasonally as in higher animals. Semen is manufactured by the gonads, so it should be secreted, -is about the only reason science can give for man's sexual activity. Tears are produced by the tear glands but should we cry all the time just for that?

About the only other mundane form of answer I have had to this question, besides reproduction, was given by a lady who had read our Lesson II of this course and thus took to being offended because it named a condition she had not remedied, but with her superiority of woman complex, had to get back at man in some way. (We are not condemning men or women, but are trying to eliminate sin). She wrote, "My mother told me man's sex excesses were only a nocturnal urge or means to cleanse his own body of disease-in other words-man has ever dumped his sex organ load into a woman's organ defiling her temple and blaming woman for every weakness and sin he wallows in."

This lady and her kind has our sympathies for her experience in the martyrdom called marriage, but why should she reason that because woman cleanses monthly her reproductive chemistry, that a man's fluid of life is only waste to be eliminated from the body. A number of people have thoughtlessly come to the conclusion that sex is a natural body cleansing process, because of its frequency among the civilized people, location in the organs of elimination and relation to the stimulation given by diet.

In the reproductive argument, science has found that the male cell or spermatozoon and the female egg or ovum unite or are fused together for development of a child embryo. Also, however, in examining the chemistry they found 40 drops of blood equal to only one drop of semen. Yet in our times when people are continually without reserve giving a pint of blood for medicine, and though the same effect of weakness is noticed after a blood or seminal loss, one escapes seeing the importance of this vital fluid that gives substance for, our brain, nerves and body tissue when conserved. Not only is the vital seminal fluid not mere tissue waste as is the urine, but also, reproduction of other beings is only a very secondary creative purpose.

The substance elaborated by the reproductive organs is first for our own perpetual reproduction or re-creation. This is the true virgin birth, how each cell of our body receives new substance from the reproductive organs to make each part born anew. Someday a race of people like angels shall inhabit the earth, and the last of the sexes having evolved out of the animal way of life, shall reproduce, each one their own virgin mother perhaps activated only by a gentle smile, a tender embrace or other purely magnetic exchange to make their own fountain of youth surge new life to all their form from the most refined human love. Not only is substance "reabsorbed," but the sexual energy is sublimated into higher activity. Man is a slave to accepting a trivial sensual pleasure for a few moments lasting, for sacrifice of an eternal ecstatic conscious-ness in God-union. The doctrine that the reproductive glands have (other-than-urine) fluid to be emptied out because of a "healthy" reproductive urge or means needed to eliminate im-purities, continually, tries to justify a tremendous and indiscreet waste of one's life fluids. Disease will only prove the result.

The appearance of sex in man and woman can be ex-plained by a pure philosophical reason. All the progress of the world has depended on sex because the soul of progress is variation. If mere reproduction were the purpose of the sexes, then only one sex would have been sufficient. God created the first man a hermaphrodite (male and female He created the first mankind) referred to as the race of Adam Kadmon in Hebrew scriptures meaning a bisexual race of man from whom later came the two part sexes. But with one common ances-tor and the same inheritance every new born person was the same in qualities to others of the race. It is by the many billions of variations in humans that progress in the human race is now evolved. Not only is the physiological evolution of man benefit-ed thru the inheritance of both sexes, but the mere association of man and woman creates ambitions and desires to impress one another in self-perfection from efforts to become attrac-tive to one another. Even in the amoeba (and other unicellular organisms) whose reproduction is by binary fission (dividing in two) which should not involve any sexual sin, yet their creative powers are regenerated by magnetic influence of other amoe-ba. In fact, our contention is that segregation of the sexes in ascetic living, as well as the so-called "right breeding" of chil-dren, is with objectionable logic and results.

As one moralist writer put it, "Daughters should be

warned against having girl friends for the first sins of maiden life are given seed in that companionship," and this homo-sexual intimacy permitted among boys only has resulted in communicating an evil mental outlook on sex. Medical officers in famous boy's schools have found that 90% to 95% mas-turbated. What makes the relations of one sex with the same sex more innocent than with the other sex? The most immoral practices are to be found in the same sex by public approval such as the tough boy's gang, men's liquor clubs, women's gossip circles, etc. Yet the association of innocent children, boys with girls, or religious monks with nuns is looked upon as unwholesome, when it should be encouraged for the effects of uplifting exchanges of electrical charges in their creative force. Education, not secrecy should be the guard against immorality, knowledge being the greater power than evil.

Aristotle is said to connect love with the doctrine of "Katharsis" or the conversion of passion general into virtuous disposition, and early Christianity took the idea further as we see their great mystic, Abba Macarius the Great, describe the gradual transmutation of fine substance of the 'soul' into still finer material of the spirit under the influence of "Divine Fire". The sublimation of the sex force and substance, though often thought of as a characteristic basis of oriental spiritual devel-opment, is seen to be recognized throughout all our religions as a creative urge that can be directed from the lower passions to spiritual realities. Birth and Rebirth are effected respectively by sexual generation and transmuted regeneration.

The purpose of the sexual organs has been miscon-strued to be for sexual union imitating the lower animals. How-ever, humans use the excuse of reproductive instinct to mean for nocturnal pleasure in extreme abuse. The human female most normally has a "very tough membrane which may some-times almost close her vagina", we now quote Elmer Keeler, M.D., and also he claims surgical operation for penetration is necessary in cases. The wedding night is associated with traditional barbaric practices of a bloody rupture of the bride's hymen to prove her virginity. Though Dr. Keeler taught semen conservation in his method of sex communion, he insists the hymen is a "troublesome and useless membrane". However, we doubt the purpose that he holds for these organs.

Nature has not made a mistake. Just like the tonsils, appendix, etc., these things that man has not found the purpose of, should not be removed, as certainly the Creator's plan had reason for them.

First the hymen shows that sexual intercourse is not natural, not in our Creator's plan for us, and who could say the bloody rape of a suffering female is a birth sanctified by God. However, medical men like Dr. Keeler claim that this hymen in females and elongated foreskin in males that makes coition a mechanically unnatural function in humans, is not hygienic. He recommends methodical stretching of the hymen (which ordinarily occurs thru cruel abuse) so it will not prevent the free exit of the menstrual blood, as well as the removal of the elongated tight foreskin early in life. Yet this is not new as the ancient Jews insisted on circumcision of the males, and in India women in their monthly periods are forbidden in the sacred temples, ever conscious of a fetid sin connected with sexual organs.

How cometh this in the holy temple of the Lord! Sin is not in sexual organs or semen. Only semen, that is wasted becomes impure. It becomes offensive by its smell warning us of the sin involved. Circumcision does not really clean out the male organ and may even encourage an even more immorally unclean life and taking women out from public contact on her physiological cleansing days does not get at the root cause of the evil condition. Whether it is the rot of male semen or the rot of the female egg causing menstruation, they are fetid signs of violation of Cosmic laws of life. The cleanliness of sex, and consequently of the entire body and mind, is dependent on sealing the organs of temptation from loss of any vital fluid, but mutilating the organs to accommodate copulation is not purity. A symptom of this is seen in certain people, who continually claim to feel unclean though having bathed just yesterday and certainly appear clean in body and clothes. No one has ever known real cleanliness and purity till the sex is free of organic sin, so the emanations are pure and wholesome to smell, touch and sight. As long as there is a rotting or disintegration of male or female seed in nocturnal emissions, spermatorrhea, masturbation, copulation or menstruation the sin will smell. Once one purifies the body through a Vitarian semen conserving diet, the excess nourishment that becomes fast rotting seminal matter will not be manufactured by the body, eliminating the cause of seminal losses including menstruation. Why be a rotten egg factory? Why should humans not have a clean fragrance about them if they are pure. It is claimed certain saints emanate delicate and delightful fragrances like that of celestial flowers, as well as emanations of light rays; in spite of sleeping on the earth (really "clean dirt") and rarely taking a full bath. Cleanliness is holiness if it means basic purity in body. This religious term, purity, is with a true ring if it means immaculate semen conservation. If one has the genuine Baptism complete, then one is not hankering for more bathing, as Baptism partakes of birth from God constantly, so one "committeth not sin for his seed abideth in him." (I St. John III:9). From this last quotation of the Holy Scriptures is clearly seen that sin is committed when the seed does not abide within one.

We do not wish to condemn; married men and women but what marriage masquerades. We quote from Dr. Keeler's course again; "Marriage is legalized prostitution. The term marriage is more offensive than the term, rape, murder, or prostitution, because it implies. all of them, and all combined are worse than either alone. The wife is the most degraded of all prostitute; a forced prostitute....When a woman has made this agreement she has made herself a legal prostitute until death or divorce. Popular prostitution, bad as it is is not as bad as the forced prostitution of marriage." Religion tells us all are born thru sin, but what are they doing about this sinful way of childbirth? Yes, to contradict this they enslave woman to the lusts of men by a corrupted sacrament known as marriage.

That woman can conceive children without any sinful act of a male is the teaching supposed to be in the always-virgin Mary giving birth to the Christ child, which is now claimed to scientifically be proven possible by actual cases in humans as well as animals who have had birth from female body alone. However death is the wages of sin, and when we are perfect we will be eternal with one body forever so as to eliminate a need for reproduction of the race. More reason against human sexual contact are the dreadful venereal diseases, especially syphilis that is to be found in the great part of our population. Prostitution is described to inflict irritations that form warts at first, later tumors and cancer appears, but most probably an erotic married couple can faster produce the same results. Beware of prolonged irritation of tender membranes the Cancer Educators tell us.

Satisfaction in sex depends on the level of consciousness of the individual. The brute man likes the tactics of the cave man who maimed his mate to unconsciousness for his lusts and many marriages come only short of this. Nor would he be satisfied with anything but excessive waste of life fluid. A higher type of man still bound to mate and giving birth to children, will get complete satisfaction in a long ecstatic sexual union without orgasm (called Sex Communion, Karezza or "coitus reservatus") which is unlike copulation that is all over in a few moments and drains the body's vital fluids. The effort for control must be greater than the desire for pleasure sought in reward though the technique of controlling the semen under all conditions can be learned by anyone. However as virginity is violated thus even the more aesthetic lovers find complete satisfaction in magnetic exchanges in embraces without resemblance to the animal procreative act. The Divine Fire of love, whether embracing individuals or God ascends like a flame purifying the mortal man to spirituality. Certainly the highest love is of God, and the Lord our only Complete Content in our search, though often the self can be transcended by influences of complementary souls, and creative virtue expressed if an object for it be found.

LESSON XII

HOW THE SEX IS SUBLIMATED

Conscious sex sublimation can be practiced by all, that is whether one lives the celibate's cloister or hermit existence or is married, i.e. with or without the presence of the opposite sex. That which makes the bodily existence of the opposite sex indispensable indicates that the lower passion is probably involved still. And by this time we should now have also sub-limated our concepts of passion. Before we have mentioned passion to indicate immoral feeling, but now that our being is gradually purged of the lower, we are becoming capable of higher passion, religious feeling or devotional ecstasy.

First let us compare the teachings on sex sublimation of H. E. Bulter, founder of the Christian Esoteric Fraternity, whose writings early in this century influenced a great number of modern cults about the inner chamber teachings on purity. Here are some notes we have copied for you from his book, "Practical Methods that Insure Success".

"The organ of generation has but two uses, the first and principle one is to generate seed for the purpose of supplying the body and brain with proper powers; the second to produce children. No one should under any circumstances, allow the slightest escape of seed, only in the case of married people when both husband and wife desire a child".

I personally knew of an instance in which a man who was retaining all the seed worked continually, day and night, for months with only one or one and one half hours rest dai-ly, which he took lying down upon a lounge and immediately taking control of the body. His mind continued active while his body laid like a clod for half an hour or more; after which the sex nature would become active in its office of transmuting the elements of the blood into life and this would continue, without any violation on his part, for perhaps half an hour, and then cease. He would then arise and go on to work much more refreshed than if he had slept twelve hours.

We do not mean to kill out all activity or feeling in the sexual organs, because the purpose of that organ is to gener-ate and transmute the seed for the use of body and the brain, and for the soul food: therefore we mean simply that you get that organ under the control of your will.

One whose nature is very active, and who experiences much difficulty in getting control, should make every effort to suppress all sexual activity, just as if the effort were to kill it out; another who has activity, but no difficulty in preventing waste of the seed, should not suppress a normal action, especially after sleep or quiet rest; for that is nature's time and method for reinvigorating the blood. We hope none will allow a depraved imagination arising from inflamed and unnatural passion to deceive them into any kind of abuse. There are two kinds of passion, each very different from the other; one imagining base and low Indulgence; the other, an energy, activity; and is entirely free from any base imaginings and desire.

If you are among the many whose vitality is low because of weakness, which renders you unable to hold the vital fluids (and the loss of these fluids is the source from which arises all lack of vitality;-many young girls inherit weakness so that as soon as they begin to generate life, they begin to lose it from this cause alone), then it is important that you concentrate all your powers in that direction, and that beginning with the first of these instructions, you follow them up with will and decisiveness. Those who have no consciousness of activity of the sex life as well as others should guard themselves and make sure that there is no waste. Many delicate ladies, who are entirely unconscious of any sexual activity or waste can by will, take control of that organ when they will discover that the absence of conscious activity has been occasioned by the continual loss of the seed generated, and as this ceases they will find themselves in possession of a great power which will tax their utmost ability to subjugate. The function of the sex organs is, to the mind and body, like that of the digestive organs to the body, their action does not mean gratification, but service . . . . . . . . while we are potent with life, there is a harmonious interchange and interblending which feeds the body, mind and soul; and when the life is exhausted, nothing remains but the memory of what has been, and the desire to find it again.

One of the causes of delight in the virginal association of the sexes, is the interblending of the positive and negative life-elements obtained from the magnetism emanating from each. The blending of these magnetisms creates life. Life is not a material substance but is a refined, subtle element permeating the whole body.

In the generation of offspring the germ is animated by the blending of the life-elements in both parents; but when the life elements blend throughout the entire body, the pleasure transcends all others that the human organism is capable of feeling. Love is a hunger of the life which produces motion, and guides the emanations to the object loved. It is a well-known fact that a person filled with life can dance about a carpeted room, and coming suddenly up to a gas burner, light it with a touch of the finger. This being true you will readily see how much of an interchange of sex life there is in a company during an evening's dance.

Truly everything is obtainable thru a chaste life, a life of self-control and everything desirable is lost by indulgence. The seventh commandment says, "Thou shalt not commit adultery." Is it possible to commit adultery? From the ordinary under-standing of the term, adultery means to adulterate with other qualities than the primary one. All know the natural impossibil-ity of two men associating with the production of a child. What could this commandment mean?

Your writer never had the physical presence of a master to train him and has arrived at the Goal without such a teacher. However, for the world, that is not enough, various types are therein represented, so we have studied the various methods by which others have attained the goal, and present them so you can see and individually learn regardless of who you are.

Here is the teaching of Yoga in the words of Swami Siv-ananda on conscious sex sublimation: "Just as the oil comes in the wick and burns with glowing light, so also the veerya or semen flows up by the practice of Yoga Sadhan (Path) and is converted into Tejas (Fire) and Ojas (Spiritual Energy). The Brahmachari (Celibate) shines with Brahmic Aura in his face...One who has perfect control over sexual energy attains powers unobtainable by any other means." Speaking of Sex Contraction of Vajroli Mudra, the Swami says: "Now there are very few people who can do this Mudra. The students, during the course of Sadhana draw water thru a silver tube (Catheter specially made) passed into the urethra. After some practice they draw milk, then oil, honey. They can draw mercury at the end and even without the help of the silver tube. Even a drop of semen cannot come of the Yogi who practices this Mudra. The Yogi draws semen up and preserves it as Ojas Shakti (Spiritual Energy). This must be done under the direct guidance of a Guru (Teacher) who has mastered the Mudra."

Now all this is true to the last statement, and we warn you that the sex fire is the most destructive fire we have. Unless you have rooted out the dietary source as well as other causes of uncontrollable passion, these instructions on internal muscular contraction or suction may only become a means to temptations in lower desires that can overcome one by this cause in organic passion. Yogis prefer the posture of sitting cross-legged in which the spreading of the legs gives greater freedom of the sexual organs which prevents tumescence in conscious transmutation thru meditation. However, tumescence (erection) is not an evil but should be controlled by the will turned off and on like an electric light with a switch. It is only when it runs wild like a loose horse and cart that it is to be feared. It is so prevalent among people in general so as to be recognized as universal. If you are not able to relax in a Yoga posture, try lying on your back drawing the legs up under one cross-legged with pillows or covers rolled under the legs to give relaxed comfort. Or one can lie limp on the back with arms thrown back over the head crossed in a circle so as to throw the chest up and keep the natural spinal curve. Thus you can practice internal contractions to insure a steady perpetual conservation of the vital fluids and experience the ecstatic regeneration of one's body after work and sleep. As it will eliminate many hours of sleep, this gained time can be employed in regenerative meditation in early morning hours (while the world sleeps) to give power also in spiritual endeavors to our greater Self in humanity.

Mother Nature has sanctified a holy rite to the "Woman clothed in the sun" in the worship (embrace) of the Holy Virgin (Mother of Life, Christ) as we explain in our book, "A Cosmic Universal Conception of Religious Living", by which we are referring to an ideal of glorifying sun bathing. Sun bathing is internal exercise of the body, and the work carried on by one's blood circulation in elimination of dead tissue and toxins can leave one completely exhausted after a sun bath as though one had done heavy labor. Regenerative meditation can be best practiced sun bathing and will counteract this weakness after one's baptism of solar light and fire.

Conscious sex sublimation can be used to invigorate one on all planes of existence. Many people spontaneously "gird up the loins" (pull a notch up on belt) when attempting any heavy work, subconsciously calling up the lower energies. Sometime while out hiking till you feel you are exhausted to the point that another step would feel too much, remember this key to all physical and mental strength, and experiment activating the sexual force through the will, which will result in an astounding renewal of vigor not only mentally but physically. New energy and will power take over the muscles as well as an alleviation from bodily exhaustion. Also this can be used to invigorate the mind, will power, Clairvoyance, and other powers leading to Divine Rapture. Finally if there is a Complete Sublimation of all lower substances of the body, one should be able to dispense with taking in any more substance in the form of food, as there would be no reason for replacement of body substance ordinarily lost in seed losses.

This exercise should be mastered alone first; further instruction than we have given on meditation will come spontaneously by prayer and when it is completely mastered it can be extended to a bisexual relationship. This rejuvenating rapture may extend to hours, and become more essential than eating and sleep in one's physical, mental and spiritual life. Do not, however, expect to inherit control from your old self to be a master in life conservation, without a period of adjustment creating a new vehicle for this which requires a sacrifice for that which is so precious.

That there is essential purity in man and woman can be seen in religious worship. Priests and monks kneel to and chant a hundred "Hail Marys" to the "mother of God," and by this devotion to the beauty of beauties they arise each time regenerated with new life. To the onlooker this is nothing but tedious monotonous chant that should tire one. Geo. Washington (a Mason) and many of the Protestants of past centuries besides the Catholics have honored Mary. While physical birth comes of the union of man and woman physically, spiritual birth is of contemplative devotional union of virgins. However, as we have tried to explain, truth is many sided, the opposites all combining in one spiritual truth. We sincerely believe in the honor and contemplation of the Virgin Mary which is a feminine principle, abstractly understood as Mother of God, Christ or Life (and thus related to the sun as its source). But the Christ was born of a male virgin if we take the Holy Bible literally. He Himself did not ever say he was born of a female virgin, and did not honor his so-called mother, saying to her once, "Woman, what have I to do with thee" Not only did he say everyone must be born again before they can enter the kingdom of God, but he called his new self, "the son of man". Yes, Christ is the son of man, of a male virgin, and not "born of a woman" as he spoke of John the Baptist. Now Mary may have been mother to the child Jesus (Matt. 1:16), who later gave birth to the Christ (Cosmic Consciousness). The lesson to be learned is that God-Consciousness is of virgin birth without multiplying bodies or changing sex. In I John 3:9, John Beloved describes the method saying the seed abideth within him who is reproduced of God, that is the sons of God are born of their own seed, with new recreated bodies.

Thus the creative substance, semen, produces the base of the blood which is called the "life of the body", and then the blood builds the body tissues and bones out of the food and air it assimilates. Oxygen makes the blood red in color and the digested chyme or food juice thins out the reproductive cell matter or semen, that becomes the egg for reproducing the various new cells of the body.

The late Mahatma Gandhi who held the vow of Brahmacharya (chastity) from 1906 to his death in 1948 said: "Maintenance of perfect health should be considered almost impossible without Brahmacharya leading to the conservation of the sexual secretions. To countenance wastage of a secretion of the sexual secretions which has the power of creating another human being is, to say the least, an indication of gross ignorance." And it is the fasting and abstinence from heavy food (besides other factors) that makes it possible for these holy men to be able to conserve their lower force for the sublime blossoming of spiritual power and moral beauty.

LESSON XIII

WHY DIFFERENT FOODS AFFECT DIFFERENT PEOPLE DIFFERENT WAYS AND THE PHYSIOLOGY OF HORMONE SUBLIMATION

"Oh, avocados don't affect me, I can eat all I want and not lose any vital fluids." "No, I can use bread and it doesn't affect me if it is whole wheat." "A little nuts don't bother me." "Don't assume that because certain foods affect you, that they will affect others. Different people are affected in different ways by different foods." These are statements I get continually from students concerning the chart on Vitarian and Passion stimulating foods in Lesson V. They think because they are not affected at the moment, that they are safe in using certain foods continually, and moreover claim I am wrong in saying that foods they like to indulge in are not good. But what makes this factor so relative among people, different foods affecting different persons different ways?

Some foods are concentrated in protein and seed elements enough to cause a fairly regenerated male body immediate nocturnal emissions. Other "border-line" foods such as potatoes, avocados, black rye bread, and other less pro-tein foods used constantly from day to day produce little or no noticeable effect on one when used in very small amounts, but rather build up a periodical excess gradually so the loss ap-pears to have no relation to the food eaten. The habit is inten-sified so that it gradually takes on the appearance of a periodic biological function that could be referred to as "menstruation" even in men. It would be just as foolish to assume that be-cause a man does not have an immediate effect from foods of excess semen-producing quality, it will not contribute to a later loss, just as it would be to assume that a woman would menstruate immediately because she ate a beefsteak, eggs or wheat germ. The loss propensity is built up gradually from day to day, and after one has forgotten about one's violation, happening even on a fast, along will come the monthly loss in woman or man unless they have degenerated to partial or complete impotence or menopause.

The onset of this periodical biological habit of elimination of excess human seed is what makes the difference between the saints of God-realization and sinners. As long as the brain substance and energy is lost in the sewer thus, one cannot have higher mental power to contact the undeviating intuitive Truth that gives one will power. This being so much more a characteristic of woman is why the Eastern Yogis so value a birth into a male body over that of a female, the male having greater ability to know by immediate feeling what is wasting their physical and mental strength and sustenance. However, woman becomes the weaker sex only because she cannot become sensitive enough to know what foods cause seminal excess, just as the more degenerate male who has lost the sensitivity of being affected by foods that affect other males of an intense vitality, youth or complete assimilative power. The importance of watching every mouthful of food escapes them till gradually they have an intolerable excess gathered to give menstruation or a heavy pollution. The large fleshy body of priests, some Yogis, and other celibates, though controlling sexual losses without living on a Vitarian mucusless diet, is not that they have transcended diet, but because the assimilative power is physiologically (thru intestinal coating and a digestive wear out) and psychically destroyed, so they are deprived of sexual vigor. Just as is the case with castration and other operations of that nature, the physical and mental degeneration or old age is not held off in a crippled assimilative potentiality. Unless intuitively perceived in rare cases, such conditions persist so the woman or the "menstruating" man has no guide to regenerate their bodies except now that we have brought out a scientific guiding chart. Of course, let me remind you that the Vitarian food chart of Lesson V is a guide, to reactions from a fairly regenerate body which has lived years on a fruit diet, fasted considerably or always lived on fruit and vegetables. A person having crippled their assimilative power through the conventional diet of much protein and starch, never cleansed completely by fruit diets and fasting, and whose glands are worn out, aged and near impotence,-will not get strong effects from moderately passion stimulating foods till they regenerate the body by fasting and fruit diets. Fasting, fruit and raw food diets are now known to restore assimilative powers in people of advanced ages, even giving them potentiality of bearing children and other physical and mental characteristics of youth they once lost.

Fasting and the fruit diet cleanses the mucous coating and cemented debris that accumulates in the intestines, tones up the digestive faculties, and takes away the excess that makes the organism refuse or be unable for protein and seed element assimilation, so that there can be greater sexual force or activity. As one ages the system degenerates, is clogged by mucus-forming grains, nuts, seed, and gelatinous foods, and these foods destroy their own assimilability. So several elder writers with gray beards are writing that sesame seeds, various alkaline grains, or even nuts do not affect the semen production, when they do not realize they have lost their assimilative power of youth as is the case of mucus-cleansed bodies that can get intense vitality from the light protein of fruits even. We have also known boys and young men who do not have seminal losses, and this in spite of the fact they ate proteins, seeds and even in cases flesh foods without any notice of effects. Not only (as we reasoned in Lesson VIII) can the state of the decay of the person's body be determined by the amount of protein he (she) needs to maintain normal-weight, but as we point out above now, certain foods clog the intestines and digestive system with vegetable starch, paste or glue, so one hardly assimilates any semen building elements to cause excess, or some digestive faculty, is so weak as not to digest and assimilate enough albuminous substances from food to produce an excess of semen (egg).

On the subject of elimination of menstruation through the raw food diet, let me quote the experiences of Miss Olga Howe as stated in MacFadden's Encyclopedia (Vol. V, page 2496). "During my experiment with raw food one year, the flow gradually lessened...I had to continue to follow these methods for two years before my system was so thoroughly strength-ened and purified that the menstrual flow ceased entirely.....On one occasion in order to prove that diet alone was responsible for this physiological change, I included cooked vegetables, butter, and milk in my daily bill of fare and in one month the menses appeared again. A few days fast and on an exclusive uncooked food diet quickly proved a remedial agent."

From the writings of Doctors T. de LaTorre, Clements, as well as the claims of various raw foodists, we are told of the elimination of menstruation and nocturnal pollutions by eliminating cooked foods. The doctrine they have is that menstruation and pollutions are caused by eliminations of waste from the body. It is true perhaps about leucorrhoea (whites) and the mucous membrane of the uterus, but the germinal cells (ovum and sperm) are not excess waste till wasted. In fact certain cooked foods of low protein and slightly starchy content such as pumpkin, squash, etc. can tend to clog, to prevent, or at least not give cause to concentrated assimilation of germinal cell building elements. The danger of cooked food is first in creating constipation which creates pressure on the prostrate in male and on the uterus of females, and breaking down the cellular construction of food, so a greater portion of the gelatinous albumin building elements are assimilated in too great a concentration. However, the greater amount of waste or clogging mucus (paste, glue, etc.), prevents rather than increases the building of germinal cells after chronic existence on the ordinary cooked diet. This is to say a good digestive and assimilative system gets sexual losses from building excess germinal cells on cooked foods, while a worn out, or weak digestive and assimilative system is clogged with mucus and waste till the sex glands are starved to impotence and the body begins to age. In India where ascetics live on a cooked starches diet (as do Western monks generally) there are many who eliminate pollutions but rare indeed are even the raw fooders here who can say they are masters of conservation. We have found mere rawfood-ism, using nuts and raw grains and seeds intensifies germinal cell excesses especially if these foods are ground into meals, pastes or butters so as to be most assimilable. Using nuts, grains, seeds and beans poorly chewed as would be the instinctive way without reading about Fletcherism, only very little in proportion would be assimilated and the pieces would give mechanical roughage to clean the intestines instead of clog them with paste.

When the microscopic cell is overfed, it simply splits into two or more parts. Overfeeding has been the encouraging factor in all organisms up to man, whose sexual activity is governed by heavy nutrition. Thru periodic fasting, the life of earthworms has been lengthened 19 times by scientists proving the theory that physiologically aging is controlled by diet which, conserves the original organism from sexual waste.

In human physiology science tells us that the plentiful absorption of sexual hormones into the blood communicates to the pituitary (the master or directing gland controlling the others) this status of excessive germinal sufficiency. Then the pituitary (which is the focal point of a person's consciousness or ego) generates pituitary hormones which regulate the activity of the germinal glands into producing reproductive cells and more hormones. Sexual hormones are said to stimulate the reproductive desires in the pituitary giving the phenomena of voluptuous imaginings concerning sex, etc., though we know this is not the case in people of higher consciousness in whom the intensity of higher spiritual activity would be the case according to the control of the master gland (pituitary) through the will. This is proven by the facts of castration (animals and eunuchs) in which the glands are removed so that there is no more manufacture of sexual hormones, and all the initiative or evolutionary progress of the castrated is arrested. The wild animal does not develop into a dangerous beast but becomes gentle to work with and in humans castration was practiced to keep the high pitch voice of a child or some other mental and physical stagnation in development. In connection with this it is noticed that the thymus is the largest endocrine gland before puberty, and after puberty with the development of the sex it degenerates, but in eunuchs deprived of the sexual endocrine secretions, the thymus continues well developed. This shows that the reproductive glands are creative agents capable of being vehicles of regeneration or whatever use we desire to put them to, though usually in the lower human consciousness, it is to waste or for lower pleasures (though designed for giving new births) and consequently gradual death takes over the organism.

The testes and ovaries produce regenerative hormones that enter a vein (not the oviduct in females or vas deferens in males) that take them to the heart and thus regenerate the blood that is pumped by the heart thru the arteries to all the cells of the body. (Please consult a reference book to familiarize yourself on these terms of anatomy). In this connection many theoretic methods of rejuvenation have been tried out by medical men, though the most illustrative for us being Steinach's vaso-ligature operation. The theory here was that old age was due to the slowing down of the genital glands, particularly the production of hormones, and Steinach had observed that if the production of germinal cells was prevented the internal or endocrine secretion became intensified, thus conveying to the organism the rejuvenating elements. The Vaso-ligature consisted in tying up the vas deferens (seminal duct) that carried the semen from the testes. The operation is said to give general improvement and rebirth of sexual vigor at first. The theory in first part is quite correct and is somewhat the thing that the ascetic attempts for in physical regeneration, but the method to carry it out is very objectionable as ignorant of the cause of sexual degeneration. It would be a "fine" thing (1) if by a mere impingement of the reproductive channel all could become regenerated physically and spiritually, so that people would age no more and with regenerated minds the earth would be a heaven, all through a mere surgical operation! Cosmic law is not that easily upset and souls will always need persistent willful effort to evolve to perfection, not a fast trick played on nature.

Steinach did not realize that the digestive system was adjusted to reproductive cell production in the conventional diet and in the pituitary control of a reproductive process. To produce regenerative hormones, a diet in life elements, vitamins and minerals, with absence of protein food and seed materials is needed but Steinach did not remove the dietary cause of excessive reproductive cell production. For various reasons his system was said to have been opposed. Your writer carried out a similar experiment that might reveal the reason they found it objectionable. Abandoning the lower tropics where fruit was abundant and going to live at super-altitudes in the Andies, one finds no fruit or even vegetables cultivated so that one is forced to live almost entirely on barley or other where fruit was abundant and going to live at super-altitudes in the Andies, one finds no fruit or even vegetables cultivated so that one is forced to live almost entirely on barley or other starchy seed protein. After the anterior 3 year period on the purifying fruit diet, the assimilative powers were intense creating an increase in the production of semen, in spite of the clogging effects of the mucus-forming pasty starches which of course in years can degenerate the assimilative capacity or deplete vital forces to nothing. However, having control over both the conscious and subconscious mind to the extent of preventing emissions and desiring any conscious abuse thru the will and muscular contractions preventing the rupture of the seminal sacs, a facsimile of the Steinach operation was duplicated.

The results were excruciating! The protein and seed elements of the diet produced excess semen building properties while the prostrate was excited continually by the pressure from the lower bowels from the constipating starches, to the point where there was no more room and the semen had filled to back up into the testes from the abdominal seminal vesicle. The testes are the most sensitive part of a male creating a dreadful pain from slight injury and this resulting pain from overcrowded semen without a willful release was a torture that would continue days on end while one went about feeling as though one had been hit in the privates. At first the rejuvenating effects were stimulated by the suppression of seminal losses, but using the ordinary diet principally of grains as is the general practice of religious celibates which builds up an excess of seminal fluid, gave results in agony, so that we can imagine why especially Steinach's method made no progress.

The formation of hormones and germinal cells in male and female is essentially the same as originally when there was only one sex. The regenerative system is near identical but the generative system for sexual reproduction is built on a struggle of opposite principles. The reproduction of human life begins with pregnancy resulting from the warring attack by innumerable male sperm bombarding female ovum till one is able to pierce the ovum, the child grows exploiting the parent to later abandon that to exploit his brethren in the world, and enter into a particular battle or lifelong duel called marriage or go to war murdering indiscriminately in the business they call life. Indeed, what a battle is such a life. Regenerative life is thus in essence, from the first cell conservation, in peace for individual, society and nations.

On one hand the male germinal cells, spermatozoa, are made in the testes containing 5,200 feet of tiny convoluted tubules which contain the mother cells from which the new germ cells obtain birth thru division. These germ cells travel thru the vas deferens into the abdomen where they are stored in the seminal vesicle. When sexual excitement is achieved to the point of breaking the seminal sacs the semen mixes with a prostrate secretion and continues down thru the urethra out of the penis. The female germinal cells, or the ova, are not produced in tubules, but close to the surface of the ovary that corresponds to the male testes. Like the sacs of the male seminal vesicle storing the germinal cells, a membranous envelope or follicle encloses the ova, but also it contains the female or follicular sex hormone that passes direct thru the walls of the follicle into the blood. When the ovum "matures", the follicle bursts open just as the male seminal sacs burst in involuntary pollutions or sexual indulgence. Now the ovum travels to the uterus thru the oviduct and lives a few hours after the arrival in the uterus either to be fertilized by a male sperm, or to degenerate and decompose to be eliminated with the entire mucous membrane of the uterus, that was prepared for the fertilized ovum, about every four weeks in what is called the menstrual cycle.

"Menstruation is, in a sense, equal to abortion," says the well-known Encyclopedia of Sex by authorities such as Drs. Willy, Vander, and Fisher. That civil marriage is legalized prostitution, that any sexual intercourse destroying the virginity or adulterating one sex with another is adultery, and now that menstruation is really abortion, are very strong statements, and possibly very repugnant to the average individual for personal reasons. We are giving a frank physiological analysis of what is overcome in the heaven life on earth by the perfected or "saved". As long as the body is overfed unnaturally there is an excess of albuminous matter assimilated that draws minerals from all the body tissues to manufacture excessive amounts of germinal cells, that may be intended for child bearing but is generally wasted in sexual abuses, menstruation and pollutions. Once the subconscious habit of losses is established after puberty, it becomes hard to eliminate unless we correct the dietetic cause and then thru conscious direction centered in the pituitary gland draw up the hormone secretions thru the body for cellular regeneration and especially cerebral renovation. Nature warns us thru the fetid smell of pollutions and menstruation that these are wrong or a "sin". Menstruation does not exist in a woman living the regenerative method of true virgins born of God. (See John 3:9). Nor does menstruation appear if women live the lower generative life like animals becoming pregnant during the lactation of each child, consecutively till she is barren, the absence of menses being normal physiologically during gestation and lactation. In this light, the so-called "celibate" or otherwise who does not completely transmute the excess of sexual energies and retain its substance, arrests the human seed in its development into a mature embryo, which is abortion, and can involve either woman or man. Men and women should develop a conscious control of the nerves and muscles governing the seminal vesicles and ovaries to strengthen them against easy rupture or bursting of the male seminal sacs or female follicle containing the ovum. After the combination of sexual endocrine hormones and pituitary secretions, cause is given to the rupturing of the seminal sacs, or the ovary follicle, thru mental endocrine stimulation in thoughts related to or involving reproduction. This is why it is said that thoughts and dreams on sexual intercourse are the same as the act. Jesus called looking at a woman with a lustful heart adultery, which we have explained to be physiologically true because voluptuous imaginings direct the pituitary glands to start the aggregation of substances and endocrine secretions to build germinal cells giving conception to a possible child that usually ends in abortion for the sake of abusive pleasure, menstruation or pollutions. Regenerative sexual sublimation is free of thoughts in acts that use and waste the human seed.

Someone has said, "Your glands are you," meaning thru our endocrine gland we mentally stimulate or create the conditions of our body. Mastery in sex sublimation precedes all regenerative processes and all physical and mental imper- fections should be overcome with it. This may not be true of eunuchs whose potentiality to change to the better has been destroyed, but there is no necessity to live on the conventional vitality-wasting diet so as to be deprived of regenerative hormones like the eunuchs because the hormones are used in reproductive cell manufacture and waste.

At present there are common fallacies among teachers of rejuvenation who say that an abundance of seminal fluid, the development of the organs and the ability to keep up a steady heavy production of germinal fluid thru seed foods (wheat germ, eggs, sesame seed, soybean products, etc.), has a rejuvenating effect on a person's body. Again let us outline the untruths herewithin. First it is not semen or ovum that rebuilds the body. The regenerative fluid, "seed" of our own body cells is produced by the endocrine glands of the gonads which is called sex hormones that enter direct into the blood stream that goes to the heart. This sex hormone or endocrine secretion is the seed for re-creating all the cells of our body in combination with various other endocrine secretions according to the characteristic need of the cells. Bone, nerve, brain, muscular, glandular, etc., tissue varying in composition need distinct endocrine secretions which are known to influence these qualities in growth. The semen and the ovum though getting the "seed" or origin as do other cells from sex hormones, also get endocrine secretions from other glands and albumen-forming protein assimilated into the blood from food besides minerals to give forth a life cell concentrate capable of evolutionary reproduction of another body. With a diet giving an abundance of seed minerals and proteins, or "albumen for egg production" an excess of germinal cells is produced.

However, this is unnatural for the higher man whose diet should be herbs and fruit, and whose unrealistically theorized human metempsychosis or reincarnations should develop into one long life superior to all animals (some of which live centuries). Each should do his part in arresting the hope for many reincarnations for one perfected life to spiritual absorption here and now. The belief of many incarnations accomplished little so slowly because the evident continual losses of conscious memory from one incarnation to another tending to a repetition of same downfalls without extremely vivid impressions of any experiences, perpetuating the general mundane misery of all. Rather than reincarnations we should say we are less worthy of God's grace.

Now summarizing, the building of an excess of semen or ovum wastes first the sex hormones and other endocrine secretions, and physiologically robs the minerals from the brain, nerve, bone and other body tissues (possibly to give each germinal chromo-some its characteristic), so that the whole body gives, degenerates and ages thru gradual depletion. Eating albuminous foods, protein and seeds, stimulates more and more germinal cell building and thus more and more sex abuse or waste, till the power to produce more hormones fails with menopause or impotence. All the reproductive development was for case of death, discontinuance of one's own being for others of no greater inherited capacity. There is still the argument that the semen is reabsorbed in the male though everyone knows the female ovum is rotted and lost. This is accrediting the Omniscient Intelligence or Law of being as being as foolish as the cat that licked a rasp file producing blood to satisfy its hunger! The semen is built from the blood concentrate of the body's essence, yet now the common theory is that the semen is used to enrich the blood and rebuild the body. Nature knows better than tear down body for semen to build and regenerate it again from the semen! In other lessons we showed how mineral deficiency, tooth decay, and other degeneration came from excess semen building. However, every foolish statement may hold the key to deepest truths. The truth here is that the reabsorption of albuminous semen into the blood could only create serious albuminuria in the already albumen-saturated blood built from a heavy protein and seed diet. In our theory of fasting to develop the technique of living without eating the body could be made to create its own food from the organic waste products of cellular decomposition. Just as the semen and ovum are built out of breaking down (aging) of all classes of body tissue, so could it be possible in breaking down of the morbid tissue when not eating, which the gonads would build into new cellular essence or hormones for regeneration, to live without loss or need of substance.

LESSON NO. XIV
ABANDONING DIETETICS


The first part of our course has dealt mostly with the use of foods of a higher life potential that rob or starve the body of the elements of the lower sensual passions, the second part of the course was instruction as to how to transmute and sublimate the new dynamic force acquired into spiritual power, and the third part (Volume III, Lessons 15 to 21) shall be more on applying Infinite Intelligence to eliminate food intake to liquids or nothing so as to give an opening for the expression of a new found unlimited power for Spiritual Life.

First, before introducing the new subjects, may I give a few points of caution and reassure you of the importance of the preceding teachings. New aspirants must not be discouraged by preliminary signs of the loss of vigor and strength when starting the vegetarian diet, the vegetarian diet, the vitarian diet, the fruit diet, fasting, after a sun bath, after a hike in the mountains, after deep breathing exercises, and other natural regenerative practices. The body's energies become so involved in carrying off waste that temporarily one is exhausted, but later preceding deep breathing one gets a dynamic breath, after a hike in mountains one grows stronger, sun bathing fortifies one's resistance to disease exercising and cleansing internal organs thru the eliminative process, fasting gives the digestive organs rest and recuperation, and the diets eliminate toxins that were formerly coming in too fast to be eliminated.

Your writer has been criticized on two points about his diet, that is even on an otherwise strict fruit diet he uses salad oil with tomatoes and recommends more food on the fruit diet. Neither of these has nay outer idealistic merit in appearance, yet this he found practical and ethical by experience alone. Returning from Ecuador, where no chemical sprays and fertilizers are used in their poverty, and trying to use the fruit on the markets of the U.S., he found the arsenic and DDT sprays and chemical fertilizers had such a corrosive action on the digestive tract that he has had to use salad oil for lubrication.

A prolonged irritation would soon cause ulceration and possibly cancers. Expert criticizers have argued the digestibility
of the salad oil is questionable, when this was not at all the
point in taking it, sugar in fruits already giving plenty of carbohydrates to make a fruitarian "fat", but the protective lubricant
split chemical compounds that have extra hydrogen atoms that
would easily combine with the active chemicals for the sprays,
etc., in fruits and vegetables so as to neutralize this corrosive
quality they have on human tissue till eliminated from the
system. Organic food from own garden do not require the oil
protection. (Later I found poisonous sprays and fertilizers the
greatest obstacle to success on Vitarian diet!)

As to eating more fruit than ordinarily on the concentrated almost waterless conventional diet, it must be remem-
bered that fruit is both food and drink. The greater intake of
pure water makes it more healthful to live on fruit.

Working in the hot sun constantly one can drink a
gallon of water in a day, so why should one not eat a watermelon a day just for the water besides other fruit for variety? A
few have joined me on the fruit diet but of course with "rational
quantity," yet they continually complain of being congested,
etc. One can eat half a small watermelon each meal and not
have a bowel movement till two days, because it all reduces to
water and one is thus constipated with no bulk to push out the
already worked over food. The reason man gets a headache,
or otherwise sick when he does not eat (fasting without preparation first with acid fruit cleansing regimen) is because the
food decomposes in the intestines giving toxins to the blood,
but when he eats again pushing the formerly consumed food
now a toxic waste out of the body it makes him feel fine. This
is man's vicious cycle of eating ever to keep the potential poisons he takes in moving so they don't poison him! So eating
more fruit is a hygienic value in cleansing the digestive tract
along with the purer nutrition without bringing in toxic fermentation problems.

On some of the more recent lessons another viewpoint
is expressed. A lady teacher of conservation writes me, One of
your readers wrote me she detests the way you dwell upon

sex, saying it was a delicate subject and should be held secret." I wrote her that only those who overcome can bring sex life out in the open and discuss it. Others prefer "darkness to Light," as Jesus says. Sinners are afraid of truth. They say they have transcended diet and sex. They have only overcome need of seeing improvement in themselves...in their own minds, though defiling their bodies at dinner tables and in bed at night, but still it is the one who reproves sin as Jesus did, that is called at fault. What they mean is they are so attached to their belly pleasures of eating and sex, that they do not want to hear or learn about anything that will interfere, no matter how much greater the merit and joy it can bring to the Spirit.

However, for those who are ready we shall do just that, their excuse being the object that we are working for in Spiritualizing Dietetics. Now that we have a real working knowledge that is power to overcome, we shall transcend diet and sex.

Joyously we cater to all. We have catered to those who think diet has much to do with our well-being, and that a fit temple welcomes the coming of the Lord within one, but now in the next volume we cater to those who "do not think diet and food are important." All the doctrines of man lead to the same theoretical objective in mind. Food is not important at all, and all is important about food! What matters here is whether you think in constructive application or use the statements as an excuse for, respectively, indiscriminate eating for pleasure and having signs of disease. The mental scientist is ever brushing off a crime of slow suicide in his eating by saying, "Ah, it won't hurt men, it's all in the mind," in spite of his miserable appearance constantly moaning because of his pleasures, and the very discriminate health eater worries himself sick thinking of what health foods he needs, what mineral and vitamin is lacking besides having his mind on disease rather than health. Both are on the wrong road, not realizing that food is unnecessary, not to be added as any help to the mortal mind and body.

Now before we go further into spiritualizing our dietetics to the point that our only sustenance is purely spiritual, we need some outside research to give us a real Spiritual foundation. In all religious or metaphysical teachings there are two paths, doctrines, or teachings. A good example of this is that of Buddhist t teachings, one being the "Hinayana," Lower Path dealing with exoteric Buddhist religious ritual and worship to gain a personal Nirvana or emancipation for miseries of further lives on earth, while the other, "Mahayana," Higher Path is not concerned with a person's own salvation but renouncing one' own welfare for efforts in salvation of others and with Omniscience as his only goal beyond the illusory concepts of mortal mind that claims the world as reality. The Upanishads of the Brahmans has the Lower Knowledge dealing with performance of rituals and other religious activities, while the Higher Knowledge, "Brahma-Vidya" is the renunciation of ritual, actions and knowledge obtained by experience of the senses for the attributeless Absolute Spirit and Omniscience.

Then studying the various Christian denominations, we find most all are concerned with religious worship of rituals, honoring saints of past Bible interpretations, and even the newer ones that pretend to have an esoteric teaching based this on astrology, hypnotic cures, occult magic in symbolisms, etc., while the doctrine of renunciation of worldly "realities" is distinct only in primitive and mystical Catholicism and Christian Science. The practice of the primitive life of Catholic ascetics renouncing all worldly pursuits, combined with the Christian Science teaching on the Infinite Mind or Intelligence, or God as the only Reality, and mortal mind based on carnal knowledge of the senses being the cause of sin and suffering, we have the identical Higher Path or Knowledge of the Buddhists and Brahmins. A student of comparative Religions finds the very same statements and truths given in Mrs. Baker Eddy's text "Science and Health" and in the various texts on the practice of Catholic asceticism that are found in Mundaka Upanishad and the Mahayana Buddhist texts which antedate the advent of Jesus as the Christ and Christian Science by hundreds of years in spite of Mrs. Eddy's exclusive claims of discovery. However, the oriental scriptures are not available usually to the western student, so he must choose a Christian source which will be more helpful for possibly being correlated with knowledge already learned on Christ's doctrine. We recommend you read "Science and Health" (available in most any library) before the next lesson. We do not expect you to agree with Mrs. Eddy's statements on diet or possibly other things but the general teaching will help you grasp the following teachings. For our purpose of understanding how man can exist without food, we first must learn what Existence and man really are. God does not merely exist; God is Existence. Man (the thinker and knower) does not merely live; Man is Life, just as Christ proclaimed He was.

## MASTER COURSE ON FOODLESS LIVING

After the Master Courses 1st on Diet, and 2nd on Re-generation, which Spiritualize the person thru a diet that gives regenerative continence, the Dietetics or sustenance can in turn be Spiritualized to become Life and Spirit, without need of tangible food.

Therese Neumann, born on Good Friday, April 8, 1898, "greatest mystic of our time," has lived 32 years without food or drink, and is an ecstatic who like hundreds of other stigmatists, bears the wounds of Christ besides direct vision of the Passion and other intimate knowledge of His life on earth, beyond the descriptions of our Holy Scriptures. She still lives in Bavaria.

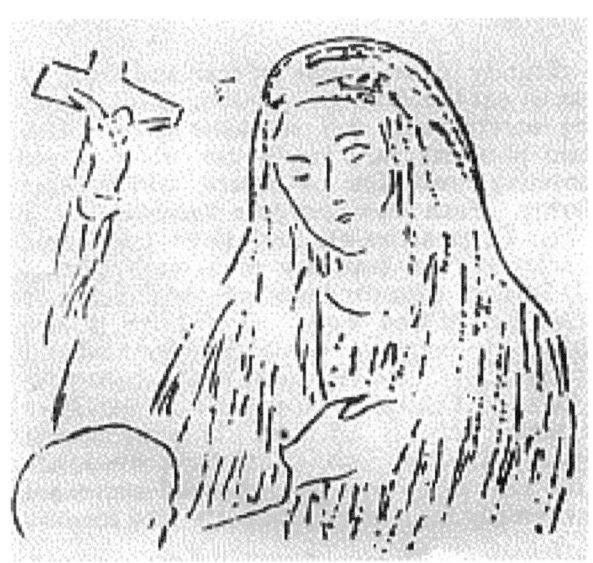

St. Mariana de Jesus, the "White Lily of Quito," pictured in Ecuadorean postage meditating on Christ Crucified, before a skull and with lily by her, symbolizing their national saint who lived 7 years without food or drink and gave her life that Ecuador's terrible earthquakes cease during great destruction in 1645.

Publisher's note: Dr. Lovewisdom realized that only by Grace can a person attain foodless living. Dr. Lovewisdom realized he was not called to this way of life and strived to perfect the diet and sexual regeneration.

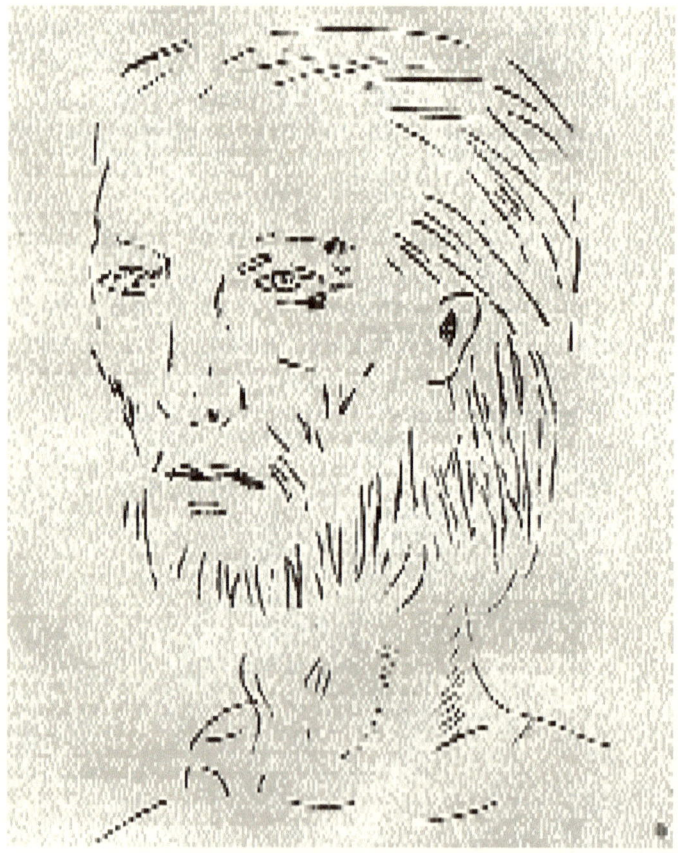

"Nikolas Von Flue, Famed Swiss Statesman, lived 20 years without food or water" is a description that Ripley in "Believe it-or-not" gave with the sketch we tried to copy above. St. Nicolas von der Flue, canonized in 1947 renounced wife, 10

children, home and went to live the Law of Christ's disciples
as an ascetic in the high Alps, giving up food. WARNING!
SHOCKING INFORMATION HEREWITHIN! NOT ACCEPT-
ABLE TO ONE IN 1,000.

## PANACEA FROM PARADISE

A TRUE CURE-ALL REMEDY FOR ALL THE SICKNESS,
SUFFERING AND SORROW OF MANKIND
Handsomely paid advertisement from the Lord God and Son.
Complete ignorance only claimed as to knowledge in the Prac-
tice of medicine by writer J. Lovewisdom, Ms. D.

Who said, "Universal cure-all? -There is no such thing." Our
greatest healer said "All things are possible with God." The
first objection to cure-alls comes from the medical doctors,
who feel they have a monopoly on the healing profession. We
observe them thru their own shortcomings. In fact, they know
less about curing disease than others, medical doctors dying
younger than other professions according to statistics.

Medicine has been described as "the art of amusing the patient while Nature performs the cure," though modern medicine cannot be laughed off so easily because in the words of Prof.... Alonzo Clark, M.D., New York College of Physicians and Surgeons, "Physicians have hurried thousands to early graves who could have recovered if left to nature," and Prof. Joseph, Smith M.D., of the same school, says, "All medicines which enter the circulation poison the blood in the same manner as do the poisons produce disease." There are hundreds of statements expressing the same truth about medicines by M.D.'s we could produce but let us dismiss all hopes in healing from medicine with the words of the great Super or Meta physician, Jesus Christ "Physician, heal thyself!" May the Lord forgive this vast homicide brought on thru ignorance. Only Truth will free man of sin.

And how did the great Meta Physician operate? First the instantaneous healings were thru God's Will synchronizing with the will to be healed and faith of the patient. Often in the Gospel He says, "Thy faith has made you whole." When he went among his own kindred, those knowing Him before His birth to God power, "he could do no miracles" and for this " he wondered because of their unbelief." Mark 6:6 However, He did not teach mere mental healing thru which the healers heal many, but deplete their own health to a miserable existence because they give own virtue or karma for healing others unworthy. "Cast not pearls to swine." The healing is only a transitory change of symptoms of disease to another. Health is accomplished if Life and Regeneration is given. "If thou wilt enter into Life keep the commandments." The Real Cure, the Panacea of Paradise is thru living the Christ-Life. For this faith in them, went forth "preaching that men should do penance" and consequently "they cast out many devils and anointed with oil many that were sick and healed them." And Matthews 17:19 shows the sure cure was in "prayer and fasting," penance doing permanently what faith could do only thru belief and the will to live the "gospel" "Do penance"! Matt. 4 Luke 8.

This vale of tears in our world of sorrow began thru the disunity or separation of man and God by disobedience to the First and Only God-Given Law in Paradise which was to eat the Forbidden Food, seeds, rather than eating only the juicy fruit. Becoming a slave to eating habit-forming earthy seeds that stimulate fleshly lusts, led to greater carnal desire and pleasures and the invention of sins to obtain pleasures thru sex abuse which begot appetite for animal flesh and fermented wine thru killing, which begot coveting possessions of others, which begot stealing, which begot lying, which begot murder, wars and all our suffering. Each new sin gave necessity for a new commandment, so the One Commandment of Paradise became the Ten Commandments and these insufficient for man's wicked ways gave need for hundreds of command-ments, and rules in the doctrines of a multitude of divided religions living in separation from God. There is only One God-Given Commandment needed to reinstate Paradise on earth, uniting all the commandments into one. This is the God Law of God Love. God Love is also Love of All, eliminating all the multiple commandments in the doctrines or religion. Christ demonstrated and taught this renunciation  of all worldly pursuits for the dedication of all one's love to God, rather than laboring for bread and meat to eat as do the worldly. This One and Eternal God Law of Complete God Love is the Love wis-dom message of our mission. This Wisdom of Love is the ba-sic teaching of all religions; it is the Cosmic Universal Religion with the unanimous membership composed of all religions. The God Law in God Love commands the God Life, this God life or Christ-Life in complete dedication to the God Law of Love is our gospel and sustenance in "VITARIANISM" or God-Life-doctrine. The following outline is our remedy for anyone's sickness and sorrows besides our Convent requirement.

CHRISTIAN SCRIPTURAL CONFIRMATION OF THE NEW DISCOVERY IN SCIENCE THAT THE SPIRIT OF TRUTH REVEALED AS THE VITARIAN WAY OF LIFE

ORIGINAL PARADISE GOD CREATED

First Scriptural God Given Commandment

God said, "Behold I have given every HERB bearing seed upon the earth, and all FRUITS, trees, that have in themselves seed of their own kind, to be your food." Genesis 1:29. Ordinary Bible translations say "tree" where fruit is indicated, because the same word was used for tree and fruit originally, just like we mean either the tree or its fruit by the word pear, or peach. Elsewhere the word to word translation says "the tree was good to eat" Douay Bible proving the word meant was fruit because one cannot eat a tree. The king James version and others have substituted phrases of explanation not found in the original scriptures to remedy this. "And He commanded him saying, of every FRUIT of paradise thou shalt eat, but of the FRUIT yielding knowledge of good and evil you shall not eat. For in what day soever you shalt eat of it you shall die the death." Of the fruit which is in midst of the FRUITS (Garden trees) of Paradise, God has commanded us: "You shall not eat of it" Gen. 2:16, 3:3 The new translation discovery reveals the long rejected hidden teaching that the food or fruit of the tree "which is in midst of Fruits of Eden meaning delight in Hebrew is the SEED of the Fruit, nuts, and other plant seeds such as grains, legumes, etc. that is yielded as a reproductive substance for plants but thru its nature also stimulates the reproductive desire to man's passion resulting in the original sin, i.e. "yields knowledge of good and evil." This is why Gen. 1:12 says, "The earth brought forth grass yielding seed after its kind and the tree yielding fruit whose seed was in midst of itself, after its kind, and God saw it was good." The sin of eating the Forbidden Food, seeds, and the resulting shame brought man the curse of being a habitual seed-eater seeking the reproductive substance because in a vicious cycle it stimulated the waste of the human seed. Man, the seed-eater, becomes the sad tiller of soil for bread and woman his slave to raise her children when God DROVE MAN FROM PARADISE saying "Behold man has become as one of us to know good and evil, and now unless he put forth his hand to partake of the Fruit of Life and live forever." ...Comparing Genesis 1:12 with 2:9 we see juicy fruits are God-Given Food of Life and SEEDS are the Forbidden Food of Death from sin and evil.

Purity of The God-Given Living Body of Man

"The lord God formed man of the dust form the earth and breathed into his nostrils  the breath of Life and man became a living soul." Genesis 2:7 "God created man in His own image, in the image of God He created him, male and female man was created." Genesis 1:27. God and thus the spirit-born man is both male and female, bisexual or asexual in certain cases. "And they were both naked, man  and woman, and were not ashamed." Genesis 2:25. "Thou art clothed with honor and majesty, who coverest thyself with light as thy garment" Psalms 104:1,2.

God-Given Labor "God made grow every fruit that was pleasant and good... and God took man and put him into the Paradise of Delight to dress it and keep it." Genesis 2:9,15

GOD-GIVEN COMMANDMENTS in man's post-paradisiacal status to check his increasing fall from Purity of Consciousness in God-Union.

"And God said: Thou shalt not have any other gods before me. Thou shalt not take the name of the e Lord, thy God in vain. Six days shalt thou labor and do thy work but the seventh is the Day of Rest of the Lord, wherefore the Lord blessed a Day of Rest and hallowed it. Honor thy Father and thy Mother. Thou shalt not kill. Thou shalt not commit adultery. Thou shalt not steal. Thou shalt not bear false witness. Thou shalt not covet thy neighbor's possessions." Exodus 20. "Thou shalt not hate thy neighbor in thine heart. Thou shalt love thy neighbor as thyself. Ye shall not eat anything with blood, neither shalt ye use enchantment, nor observe times. Ye shall not round the corners of your heads, hair neither shalt thou cut the corners of thy beard", Lev. 19:17, 18, 26, 27. "Stand now with thine enchantments, the astrologer, stargazers, the monthly prognosticators, shall not deliver themselves none of these shall save thee" of Isaiah 47:12-15 explains forbidden enchantments. Also see Daniel 1:20. "He that killeth an ox is as if he slew a man For by fire and sword will the Lord plea with all flesh, atomic fire and war, and the slain of the Lord shall be many. They that sanctify themselves and purify themselves in the garden behind the tree in midst, Forbidden Food eating swine flesh, mouse and abominations shall be consumed together, saith the Lord" Isaiah 66:3, 16, 17. This is fate earned by flesh eaters and killers. "Daniel purposed in his heart that he would not defile himself with any of the meat and wine which the king drank...Let them give us vegetable food to eat and water to drink" Daniel 1:8,12.

PARADISE REINSTATED
The Christ-Life in Vitarianism

Jesus said: "If thou wilt enter into Life keep the commandments." And the first scriptural God-Given commandment asks us to eat the fruit of Life rather than the seeds that bring degenerative lusts and death. For commemoration of Him or His sake we are to drink fresh juice of grapes in which the seed is separated from the grape blood. In the Holy Eucharist Jesus said, "Drink ye all of this. For this is my blood of the new covenant which is being shed for many. Amen, I will not drink henceforth of the fruit of the vine until the day when I shall drink it new with you in the Kingdom of God." Juicy fruit is the ONLY FOOD Jesus directly told us was to be eaten in His Government or Kingdom of Paradise "Heaven". That drinking wine "new" means fresh grape juice we are assured by Isaiah 65:8, saith the Lord, "As the new wine is found in the cluster, and one saith destroy it not "fermenting", for blessing is in it." Praising John the Baptist, the Bible says: "For he shall be great before the Lord, and shall drink no wine nor strong drink and he shall be filled with the Holy Ghost." and in Luke 7;33 we find he "came neither eating bread nor drinking wine." The true Lord's Prayer, Rheims Version, Matt. 6:11 says: "Give us this day our super-substantial bread" and Christ has explained "I am the living bread that comes down from heaven" in John 6:51, Jesus said: " My food is to do the will of Him that sent me, that I may perfect His work." John 4:34 " Man liveth not by bread alone but by every word of God." Luke 4:4; "Labor not for meat that perisheth, but for that which endureth unto Life Everlasting." John 6:27; "And seek not what you shall eat and what you shall drink." Luke 12:29; "Take heed to yourselves lest perhaps your hearts be overcharged with surfeiting and drunkenness and cares of this life." Luke 2:34; "It is the Spirit that quickeneth, flesh profits nothing....The words I have spoken to you are Spirit and Life...I am the bread of Life: He that cometh to me shall not hunger and he that believeth in me shall never thirst...He that believeth me hath Life Everlasting." John 14:6. "Do penance that you all shall not likewise perish." Luke 8:3. The Way was demonstrated in His 40 day fast and recommendation of Fasting and prayer to support Faith to cancel sins.

Throughout the Scriptures from the First Book of Genesis where the ONLY GOD-GIVEN FOOD was the FRUIT FOR LIFE forbidding the eating of the seed or FRUIT FOR DEATH for which man was driven out of Paradise to the very last Chapter in Apocalypse where it gives the REQUIREMENTS FOR ENTERING THE CELESTIAL CITY OF GOD, STATING: "Blessed are they that do the Lord's commandments, that they may have the right to the Fruits for Life, and may enter the gates into the city." besides at the Climax of Christ's Evangelic Mission at the Last Supper where Jesus commands for His sake we drink of the fresh fruit with seed extracted,...the only food that God ever permitted in Paradise, Celestial City of God or God's Kingdom in Christian Scriptures was the Fruit of Life without using the Fruit-seed of Death. With the use of the degenerating passion inflicting seeds, the one commandment of Paradise had to be multiplied into ten commandments, and then onto hundreds. Laws without Life are nothing. God-Life manifest in God-Love thru obedience of God Law.

PARADISE REINSTATED

Celibacy For God's Government

"There is neither male nor female. For you are one Christ" Gal 3:28. "For to be carnally minded is death; but to be spiritually minded is Life and Peace." Romans 8:6. "There are eunuchs who have made themselves eunuchs for the kingdom of heaven", Matt. 19:12. "They shall be accounted worthy of that world and the resurrection from the dead, shall neither be married nor take wives, neither can they die anymore", Luke 20:35. "And for raiments why are you solicitous," Luke 6:28. "Is not Life more than food and the body more than raiment" Matt. 6:25. "These are they who were not defiled with women; for they are virgins...have not defiled their garments and they shall

in white because they are worthy." Apoc... 3:4, 14:4. "Whosoever is born of God does not commit sin, because his seed
abides in him and he cannot sin, because he is born of God.
In this the children of God and the Children of the devil are
made known," I John 3:9. Here John in the Christ Spirit gives
celibate seed-conservation as the key factor in the God-Born
man. This clearly exposes the Old Testament "patching up"
of violations of holy purity by giving sin offerings as devilish
bargaining with God for exceptions to commandments against
sex defilement, perverting the Word of God to accommodate
the weakness of the flesh and covering up the symptoms of
sin rather than elimination of the hidden sin. In one sentence
John gives the law that chapters of the Old Testament were
written seeking exceptions such as: covering up nakedness
as shameful while Jesus says it is lust within the heart and of
the eye that sins scandaleth (see Leviticus 18 and Mark 7:21),
giving sin offerings after cleansing and segregation of seven
days of persons and objects touched by the seed for copulation when sex is wasted or there is any seed loss (Lev. 15),
segregating the menstruous woman rather than eliminating the
fetid sin of menstruation by application of the first paradisiacal
law with man's uncleanliness in sex-seed losses thru the pure
Paradisiacal diet (Gen. 2:16;17, 10:14; Ezek. 44:7,9), and that
the unmarried adultery is guilty of shedding blood more than
the same horrible prostituting that goes on under the rite of
marriage (Ezek. 23:45; Exceptions (i) in Deut. 21:14; etc.)

Think not that one can overcome sin of losing one's
seed by giving a priest two turtles and two pigeons as Moses
bargained with God! The Law is to conserve the seed: eat no
seed and waste no seed. Here on earth man is suffering from
disease in a worse hell than religion pictures but man happily
goes on sinning to the day of death.

Restoring Paradise Thru Fruit Culture

"And I saw a new heaven and new earth...and He showed me
the holy Celestial City of God... in the midst... was the Tree of
Life bearing twelve fruits, yielding its fruit every month" Apoc.
21:1,10; 22:2. "I create new heavens and a new earth.. and
they shall plant vineyards and eat the fruit of them," Isaiah

65:17,21

by LIFE IN THE CHRIST KINGDOM or under God's Government the Paradise of Life Everlasting can be realized within all.

"For unto us a child is born unto U.S.A. son is given and the
Government shall be upon his shoulders and his name shall
be called Wonderful, Counsellor, the mighty God, the Everlasting Father, the Prince of Peace. Of increase of his government and peace there shall be no end... They shall not hurt
nor destroy in all my holy mountain for the earth shall be full
of knowledge of the Lord. He is despised and rejected of men;
a man of sorrow. He was wounded for our sins. And made his
grave with the wicked... because he had done no violence,
neither was any deceit in his mouth...when Thou shalt make
his soul an offering for sin. The work of the righteous shall be
peace; and the effect of righteousness, quietness and security
forever. The dead shall live together with my dead body shall
they rise (resurrect). Thine eyes shall see a king in his beauty,
they shall behold that the land is very far off. Before me there
was no God formed. I, even I , am the Lord and other than me
there is no saviour. Thy first fathers hath sinned and thy teachers have transgressed against me. Therefore, I have profaned
the princes of the sanctuary."-Isaiah 8:6, 11:9; 53:3-10; 32:17;
26:9;33:17; 43:11,27. The Lord said, "I create a new heaven
and a new earth... There shall be no more thence an infant of
days nor man that hath filled his years (child-bearing nor old-
age)...they shall plant vineyards and eat the fruit of them.. they
shall not labor in vain nor bring forth trouble... The wolf shall
feed together with the lamb  and the lion shall eat straw like
the bullock (Universal vegetarianism)," Isaiah 65. Behold the
day comes saith the Lord that I make a new covenant... I will
put the Law in their inward parts and write in their hearts this
law... And they shall teach no more every man his neighbor
and brother, for they shall know me,"-Jeremiah 31:31

        The Sermon on the Mount of Jesus gives the foretold
teachings of Peace in the new Christ Kingdom, loving all,
blessing those that abuse us, giving to those who demand of
us, doing good in return for evil, returning forgiveness for
The Sermon on the Mount of Jesus gives the foretold teach-

ings of Peace in the new Christ Kingdom, loving all, blessing those that abuse us, giving to those who demand of us, doing good in return for evil, returning forgiveness for condemnation, living in the world but not letting the world live in us. Christ's REQUIREMENTS FOR DISCIPLES desirous of Life Everlasting are renunciation of wife, father, mother, children, brothers, sisters, other worldly relations and friends, one's worldly life pursuits, and all worldly possessions, for which he assures one will receive one hundredfold in God's Kingdom. (Mark 10, Luke 14, Matt. 29). The nature of the SECOND COMING OF CHRIST IS explained: "The Government of God cometh not by observation, For lo the Government of God is within you... as the lighting that lighteneth from under heaven shineth unto the parts that are under heaven; so shall the son of man be in his day" Luke 17:21 Matt. 24:27. Our God-Love must be raised to spiritual illumination to realize Christ's coming within, and universally. "Unless a man be born again of water (fasting) and Holy Spirit, he cannot enter the Kingdom of God." "I have yet many things to say unto you but ye cannot bear them yet. Howbeit when the Spirit of Truth is come, He will guide you in all Truth," John 16:12. Let us resurrect Living Christ on earth!

Lesson XV

COMMON FOODS ARE HABIT FORMING DOPE: FOOD IS NOT LIFE GIVING

In the first Chapter of this course we give the statement from Chapter 1:29 of Genesis of the Bible,-"And God said: Behold I have given every herb bearing seed upon the earth and all trees that have in themselves seed of their own kind, to be your meat (food)". As we read thru the story of Eden we find no indication that man ate herbs or grass in Paradise. It is evident that the fruit and herbs were the only foods permitted as food on earth for man by commandment of God, but in the ideal state of Paradise man eats only fruit. We have extolled the properties of fruit as a perfect food, conserving man's strength because it is ready for assimilation when eaten while other foods need twice or three times as long time to digest, and thus remaining longer in the body, other foods begin to decompose into toxins that begin to poison the body before they are eliminated. The vegetables seemed to be an emergency food should man wander elsewhere on earth from his fruit paradise.

Herbs were not pleasant in taste and appeal at first, but man cultivated them, learned to cook them and soon found he could not get along without them, not because he naturally liked them but because he got the herb habit. Anyone who has lived on fruit for years can tell you that eating vegetables is n acquired habit and that vegetables have an inorganic or earthly taste. We know the minerals in the vegetable sap are conduced to the leave to become organic through the sun's energy, that material of the vegetable roots, stems, etc., are partly inorganic matter, and that ripe fruit is the only completely organic food having finished the solar manufacture of life cells. To most vegetarians it may be startling to learn that all herbs are not natural, but habit forming...drugs, similar to those used by drug fiends, in cases. However, the properties of these medicinal vegetable drugs in our common foods are only recently discovered in effects and labeled "Health Food" to be used innocently by doctors who recommend drugless healing and natural diet. Now before there is any misunderstanding, we are going to reaffirm that much worse are flesh, fish, fowl, eggs, dairy products, beans, grains, nuts, seeds, spices, etc. But these vegetables are not so health-giving because they are natural food, but because they are so powerful in counteracting or neutralizing the effects of the heavier albuminous, starchy, acid forming diet of nuts, beans, grains, etc.

One of the most thought of salad vegetables is lettuce. It is a good alkalizer to balance the acid-forming bread, nuts or animal proteins, unless one prefers a little stronger alkaloid drugs such as found in Alka Seltzer, coffee, Coca-Cola, or alcoholic drinks. Lettuce contains a soporific called "lactucarium," a harmful alkaloid narcotic made from species of the plant and used as a substitute for opium. In Ecuador your writer found the lettuce leaf tea given to infants to make them sleep if they cried and were restless, when they did not use poppy (opium) leaves. From personal experience and that of friends, I found that although the juicy fruit diet requires only 3 hours sleep, ordinary vegetables require 6 hours sleep, and with mainly lettuce in the diet one finds 8 hours may leave one still drowsy. Plants in the lettuce family and others with bitter alkaloid tasting milk (escarole, endive, dandelion, etc.,) though lesser in effects in cases are of similar habit forming effects,... things we learn to like for health's sake that later one cannot do without.

Similar effects we have obtained from the potato diet. Potatoes are a much better food than animal substances, grains, beans nuts, and will cure ailments caused by these foods, but that is for its qualities of counteracting acid conditions of sickness from such foods. We did not find them a good permanent food for man being to another extreme in properties of one kind while otherwise too heavy a food. Potatoes contain the narcotic alkaloid, "solanine," that gives potato poisoning. In the High Andies while exploring, the only food other than grains we could find at ranches was potatoes, and many times being seed potatoes or slightly greened they leave one in a mental sopor, besides the ordinary properties, especially of baked potatoes used with skins, making one sleep more. The potato and tomato plants like that of the nightshade are poisonous to animals, tho tomatoes are not more soporiferous than some other vine fruits, they seem to have a habit forming effects on some vitarians and fruitarians making it difficult to be without them.

Not only do onions, leeks, and garlic contain soporific substances that are so habit forming as to be universally in demand by raw foodists and vegetarians who do not have access to other alkaloid vegetables, but they have irritating oils that affect the tender membranes of the genitals for which reason we definitely discriminate them as passion producing foods. In the same classification are mustard greens, turnips, etc., that contain the irritating oil of mustard besides soporific substances. Then there are the oxalic acid vegetables such as spinach of all varieties, beets, chard, etc., that also create a minor irritation that is very noticeable if they are pursued as a diet. Root vegetables are especially known to have a minor stupefying effect or weakening of deep mental function so as to be banned by some religious groups, because they bring in inorganic earthy matter that make the body energies center their action in the lower digestive organs.

In general, all vegetables dull the brain and produce enervation because they require an elaborate digestive process in the intestines, robbing the brain of blood and oxygen if not drugging it. Fruit was the only solid food intended for man's digestive system and it is nearly immediately assimilable without hours of digestive labor. In general, all substances that are the hardest to give up are the most poisonous causing the body to make the severest adjustments to withstand them. We were drugged into the eating habit. Abandoning fruit, man formed the herb habits which led him form the milder narcotic herbs called vegetables to leaves of tobacco, tea, etc., besides the use of the narcotic seeds of cocoa, coffee, etc., which enabled man to withstand effects from the use of acid forming foods such as grains, nuts, beans, and animal proteins. All our study of dietetic medicine is no more than the knowledge of chemical magic, a side show entertainer demonstrates when he pours together two or more deadly poisons (which unknown to the public neutralize the effects of each other) and swallows them without serious after effects. Recently a wealthy California man, eating the conventional acid-forming diet neutralized by the alkaloids he got in drinking wine and chewing tobacco to his last day, died at the age of 103 years. The diet of natural healers is only an imitation of the same method, combining alkaloid containing vegetable salads in right proportion with acid-forming nuts, grains, beans and other seeds so that the body poisoning or disease producing foods are neutralized. We were drugged into disease by inexperience with the use of correct proportions to neutralize the effects of each, and we drug ourselves back to health by milder poisons and accurate proportions seems to be the hidden theory. It is about time we turned from the magic show of neutralizing poisons we are addicted to, to the use of the pure perfect food intended for man that would free man's energies from the lower physical processes so he could develop mentally and spiritually. Mental and spiritual giants cannot be expected from a race of food dope fiends.

In the East they say the subtle vibrations or emanations of the body become more harmonious, pleasant and even fragrant as one lives on spiritually sublimating food. It is no wonder that the outer vibration of a body is putrid if the inner is a grave for rotting carcasses besides a minor alcohol distillery. A vegetarian overcomes some of this tho still as in the ordinary in the regenerative organs there is the stimulation that wastes the reproductive cells giving the organs especially besides the blood and perspiration a fetid emanation. The Vitarian diet of fruits and vegetables with the accompanying regimen of conservation  (of semen, menses) eliminates offensive odors from the sperm or egg cell rot in the body and the taste in the mouth immediately after sleep is not disagreeable with an urge to vomit at the mention of an early breakfast. However, it is on the strict diet of juicy fruits that the taste in the mouth is sweet immediately after sleep, the perspiration with ultraviolet life rays repels, insects rather than attracts them as is seen in herbivorous diets where gnat flies attack the eye secretions (note in horses, cows as well as man), and the residue on the genitals is not only inoffensive but at times fragrant and sweet. The later test to determine the status of one's blood thru nature of what is eliminated by the kidney from the blood as something of superfluous or injurious assimilation can be made directly in Yoga posture "Hala Asana" without any artificial equipment. Needless to say the taste is putrid if the body chemistry is putrid with starches, proteins, etc., decomposing and poisoning the blood. That bitter alkaloids deaden the nerves and reach the brain will be known because instead of going thru intestines with no effect the (alcohol, tobacco, lettuce and bitter vegetables) give this same bitter residual elimination from the blood as found in the narcotic food. Acid forming foods give the repulsive uric acid. Only on the juicy fruit diet is the taste sweet after sleep or almost  a nectar when the diet is mostly sweet fruit. Yogis speak of the sweet nectar of immortality dribbling from the palate in God-Rapture in which the lower energies are sublimated. The fruitarian with sweet nectar in his blood as the only possible "impurity," experiences this dribbling or effervescence of energy throughout the body, a lightness described sometimes as walking on air, and a powerful bliss in his mental activity, which opens the doors to spiritual nectar also.

However, even the living on semi-liquid diet of fruit we do not propound as the supreme goal in perfect living. We are giving you the various stages to perfection according to the experiences we consider spiritually advanced and it can be also compared to mythical and legendary stories of early man.

Legend, as well as present claims, tells of men dwelling in high places who needed nothing but air charged with solar energy to sustain themselves. Baggat Iran referring to this wrote, "During that time it was common to find men and women who were thousands of years old. In fact, they did not know death. They passed from one accomplishment to higher attainment of life and its reality. They accepted Life's true source and it released to them its boundless treasures." (Life and Teachings of the Masters of the Far East, V. II) Long ages pass and in time this man began to use rain water (just as some today say Himalayan masters exist on snow). Somewhat in the image of Creation, thus man's eyes were blue like the sky, his hair golden like the sunshine and with blonde or transparent complexion. The Hyperboreans, according to Greek tradition, were god-like men who lived in their high mountains, who first had lived lifespans of thousands of years on air and sunshine as their only nourishment, and later were found living exclusively on fruits. This tradition is true not only of Greeks, but in other regions such as told of Himalayan masters, the lost white race of Pre-Inca masters of the high equatorial Andies and a blonde people in Africa.

But to get a better idea of what physical man really lives on we need only look again to the Genesis legend. Man does not live because he eats food, nor was the Garden of Eden given to man to keep him alive, but it was and means Paradise of pleasure. Fruit was given for innocent pleasure, just as parents give sweets to children not as food. Man lives because "God formed man of dust of the ground and breathed into his nostrils the breath of life and man was a living (animated) soul." It does not say man lived because God gave him fruit or food to eat, but because he gave him the breath of life. It is in the high altitudes that one feels God's breath of life, winds taking one's breath away and then filling one's lungs with a blissful solar power from sun-electrified air, naturally blowing this breath of life into one. In the East, Yogis do it through muscular breathing exercises, and Western mystics naturally assimilate spiritual force from the air through religious deep-breath rapture. So it is for this "Heliovora" status transcending even the herbivora and frugivora stages that this third volume of SPIRITUALIZING DIETETICS is mainly dedicated, explaining, of course, the methods of transition (Heliovora is a term we used in No. 17 E.Y.L. of Nov. 5, 1948 to denote living on solar light energy).

However, to get a final firm foundation for even our Heliovora conception, it is necessary to first understand that Life is not energy as ordinarily spoken of, but rather Life is the All Pervading Intelligence found everywhere. Certain mystics in various religions, stop breathing for hours and days in Divine ecstasy (See Chapter VI in your writer's Life story for a personal account), and Yogis permit themselves to be buried long intervals without air to live afterwards. The news reports of July 26, 1942 gave an account of a Yogi who was buried six months in which his beard did not grow, clothes were eaten by white ants, which he explained possible through stopping mental action and other involuntary body functions. A forty day live burial is a common feat demonstrated by certain Yogis. If merely breathing were living, then they would have died and decomposed. Life is the Supreme Being, present every place underground, on earth and in the heavens, by which we live and have our being. We do not live because of substance or solar energy, a sick man dies in spite of foods and air. This is why we recommend the study of the teachings of Mary Baker Eddy (there are hundreds of others giving some principles less known) available to all.

So in the Words of Mrs. Eddy let us review understanding of the Life Principle, "The fact is that food does not affect the absolute Life in man and this becomes self-evident when we learn that God is our Life In that Perfect day of understanding we shall neither eat to live nor live to eat.....The test "Whosoever liveth and believeth in me shall never die!" not only contradicts human systems but points to self-sustaining and eternal Truth... The best interpreter of man's needs said; "Take no thought for your life, what ye shall eat and what ye shall drink...The divine Mind (Life) maintains all entities from a blade of grass to a star, as distinct and eternal Soul is synonymous with Spirit, God, the Creative governing infinite Principle out-side of finite form, which forms only reflect..The sinless joy, perfect harmony and immortality of Life, possessing unlimited divine beauty and goodness without single bodily pleasure or pain constitute the only veritable indestructible man whose being is spiritual. Death can never hasten this state of exis-tence for death must be overcome, not submitted to, before immortality appears... Nothing is real and eternal, nothing is Spirit, but God and His Idea. Evil has no reality. It is neither person, place nor thing but Simply a belief, an illusion of ma-terial sense. It is unreal because it presupposes the absence of God, the omnipotent and omnipresent. Every mortal must learn that there is neither power nor reality in evil. Mind, not matter, is causation...The realm of the real is Spirit." (Unquote)

What a beautiful teaching! Here are words of Wisdom from Christian teachings identical to the Higher Doctrine of Buddha and of Yogis, the same material that oriental scriptures existent hundreds of years before Christ came, for overcoming the mortal status of being and worldly illusion, "Samsara and Maya." With Mrs. Eddy there were healings demonstrated for her belief, while in other great teachers there have been vari-ous demonstrations for their work in absolute dedication to this principle. Miracles (so-called) are a matter of Grace, but such is not necessary to prove one's principles. However, teaching certain principles we should not contradict them for our own mortal human convenience.

Thru spiritual inspiration Mrs. Eddy said, "To cure a bodily ailment every broken moral law should be taken into account and the error be rebuked" (page 382, Science and Health). She has been very right also in saying the "Laws of matter are nothing but false beliefs," "that disease is the result of education" and attributes sin to mortal mind only but as all religions agree, our physical and spiritual well-being depends on living in God's moral commandments. Christian Science affirms, "Matter is impotent." Of course, we are very grateful to the great humanitarian aid Christian Science has put forth opposing the use of drugs and poisons for curing disease, be-sides condemning the use of tobacco and alcohol. But certain Yogis have been currently proving publicly in the U.S. the impotence of matter by swallowing glass, eating poisons, walking on fire and piercing body with nails. However, all are not Yogis able to demonstrate powerful mental control, nor do these Yogis do this constantly in same way man eats, drinks or smokes. Some get by using tobacco for a 100 years, and if they live alone they are the only ones who fight its poison. But eating animal carcasses other lives are destroyed. The moral law of not killing must be taken into account, just as Mrs. Eddy indicates but disregarded in practice so that her death-causing practice in eating bound mentally to need of using slaughtered carcasses as food gave like results in her death. Eating rich foods giving sensual passions also sins in personal adultera-tion that seeks to conquest others in adultery. Yes, matter is impotent, because it is His moral law, His word or teaching that gives us power if believed to the extent of a living practice of these principles. Rather than necessitating slaughter of a pig, cow, etc., one should know the dead carcasses are impotent, dead, powerless to help one and a serious sin against Life. The consuming  of the carcasses or any animal proteins (eggs and milk products) imparts to man's body the forceful bestial magnetism that soon penetrates his being overcoming the psychic impressions with the lower animal passions and in-stincts. How can one violate or cancel life in other beings and yet be Life by which all beings live!

If one's mind bases its life strength and power in rich nourishing meals of bread, beans, macaroni and cheese, etc., it shows we do not live on the spiritual plane of Divine Mind in which case theory and practice should attribute our existence to a self-sustaining Life Intelligence. If these foods are import-ant to our well- being, then they should be given to the starving millions who do not understand this to save live, rather than wasted on our  belly pleasures. This is living the Science of Christ, rather than the arguing of defense for our mortal de-sires.

Mrs. Eddy gives the case of a person who took up the vegetarian Graham system of curing dyspepsia, living on a slice of bread daily only. He was given up to die, but at that point "Christian Science saved him." Thru it he reasoned eat-ing animal flesh could not over power him if God had dominion over all. God never made dyspeptic and returning back the conventional diet he was cured.

But this is no argument for a Scientist to eat meat causing sin in slaughter which should be rebuked as she taught otherwise. She admitted the food has no power in cure, but the moral and mental sin gave us disease. There is much truth in her statement, "With rules of health in the head and the most digestible food in the stomach there would still be dyspeptics," but it would be foolish to conclude that the moral teaching of Christ and the belief that God is sustainer, can thus be discarded. The cure of the mentioned dyspeptic has no bearing on food taken, but for accepting Christ as the sustainer and physician in belief. But belief in many things can cure. Mrs. Eddy gives the case of Sir Humphrey Davy curing paralysis in a patient by merely putting a thermometer in his mouth, the latter thinking it a remedy becoming well only thru mental belief. Giving some body some impressive remedy, some lauded "Health" food or diet, they say they are cured, but let us not give potency to matter. Only Mind Omnipotent can cure or do anything, we should credit and thank God for the cure or action and not the powerless material things. Simple mental cures in some remedy of belief or medicine often are valueless many times, showing them to be in the plane of chance and change, but thus gives growth to our worldly science of speculation and confusing contradictions.

Throughout the various new teachings of the Science of the Mind, it is emphasized that "Food is not important." This we believe, teach and try to practice by giving the least importance to food values, gradually breaking hold that matter and false notions about it had on us before. Mrs. Eddy foretold the presentation of this new information on page 388 in Science and Health, admitting that in her day without a "clear comprehension of living Spirit" it would have been "foolish to venture beyond her understanding...to stop eating," though in "that perfect day of understanding we shall neither eat to live nor live to eat." Besides our own progressive experiments we shall give the facts on cases of others living without eating so as to pave the way to a greater acceptance of a foodless "Heloiovora" existence. Knowing that food does not affect the Absolute, that only thru the Power of God do we live, keep well and perform any actions we will not give power mentally to pleasure stimulating foods, bitter drugs, and remedies to shift us from one illusion and sin to another.

"Vitarianism" is a technique for the "resurrection into Life" or the conquest of the spiritual plane of living. The Christ called himself the Life, or "Vita," and thus we have taken the Universal Life Intelligence as the devotional goal of living.

There is a reason for the new term: Vitarian we say rather than Christian, because Christian unfortunately is unanimously used for our greatest killers besides other sinners while those in Christ should be freed of sin and to discriminate from these confusing manifestations of principle by Vitarianism we wish to give our Christ's teaching on the Eternal Universal Life Principle which also is the essential teaching and moral code in other religions such as Buddhism, Brahmanism, etc. Rather than a sectarian teaching, a Supreme Being comprehended as the Life Principle of the Universe would be taught to avert rejection, prejudice and religious battles. Accepting "Life Omniscient" as the Allah, Tao, Spiritual Buddha and Christ of the Universe, all mankind can be united under one Godhead for God's Kingdom on earth.

Vitarianism means Life respecting and Life conserving, which includes conservation of all living sentient beings, wild life and forests, eating no more than herbs and fruit as a diet and sublimating rather than wasting regenerative life fluids for abundant Life force and intuitive spiritual knowledge. "Vegetarian" having origin in life and quickening force also, today does not convey meaning other than eating vegetables. Our fruit and herb reform was for a transition from belly-living to spiritual-living, "Spiritualizing Dietetics" However, Real Vitarianism is Spiritual Consciousness attributing our existence only to Life Omniscient, Omnipotent and Omnipresent. This Life is not obtained by conserving living beings (vegetarian), living on live foods (raw foodist), eating only perfect food (fruitarian) or absorbing nourishment from air of sunlight (Breatharian or Heliovora), though these are progressive steps to Absolute Vitarianism which recognizes only the Supreme Spiritual Intelligence as our only Life essence, Absolute Vitarianism is an Insight and Recognition of Spiritual Reality by living this Truth.

LESSON XVI

"AND THE SPIRIT OF GOD FORMS MAN OUT OF THE VAPOR AND EARTH ELEMENTS IN THE AIR, THRU THE BREATH OF LIFE TO MAKE MAN A LIVING SOUL"

To understand how man is made, and now he gets his strength, certainly science has no explanation. Dr. Alexis Carrel, famous contemporary surgeon said, "The science of man is still too rudimentary to be useful. The illusion of the mechanist of 19th century, and the childish physical-chemical concepts of the human being have to be definitely abandoned" in "Man, the Unknown." Perhaps the ancients can tell us, since their data in scriptures have proved them thru the centuries instead of having to be rejected every year for new discoveries. Seeking "how is man's body made," if we understand that time is not a Cosmic Reality, the same question can be understood as "how was man made" and how will he always be made.

In Genesis 2:7, it says man was made from the dust of our planet earth, meaning he is made of invisible earth elements in the air, which are made living substance of the body by a life-giving spark in the breath of life that makes man a living soul. This can explain how life started on earth. Yogis in the East are able to materialize more than one body out of the dust or earth elements in the air so as to be seen at two places at once. Understanding this it is not difficult to understand how man migrated from other planets to people the earth, by materializing bodies like he had on another planet on earth, even without theories about space ships. This form of reproduction is the only true immaculate conception of new soul dwellings, by which "there will be no more infant of days and man that hath filled his years" (Isaiah 65) which happened when God put Adam on earth, when Christ ascended resurrected from the dead, and when anyone knows true spiritual or God-Birth on earth. This is Birth in the God Image or Christ Principle on earth.

But how did man continue to live on earth, though not in the God Image fallen to mortality? He lived the same as before from the Breath of Life, though less abundantly and this breath is what man is formed out of today. From the gaseous and vaporous earthy substance in the air, the body is built and animated by the Power from Breath of God or Life Everlasting. Notice why we clarify the simple scriptural statement so it will not be taken that some energy in the air is the Life Everlasting, but rather thru breathing we get cosmic energies and substance from the air for the power of animation. The Life Everlasting or God goes on immortal in the God Image always, whether or not man breathes, so mere breath is not Life, though the Cause of breath, the Cosmic Breath is the Divine Life of all things eternally. To explain this we need only observe that all animation can be suspended completely to the absence of breathing even, but Life can reinstate function to a body. We told of the Yogi being buried for six months with no air who lived again, Jesus resurrected his body from death in a grave in three days, your writer was without breathing or detectable heart beat for one day in a spiritual ecstasy to be taken for dead but he resurrected thru an intense will to live, making it impossible to remain dead in spite of advance decay of body in the tropics, and in recent years animals have been reinstated to animation in spite of being frozen for unknown centuries in Siberia. They all stopped breathing not because the life of them was destroyed, but because breath was halted. Breath does not give or produce Life Everlasting, though Life is the Cause of Breath and all things, Life being another name for Omnipotent God.

Yet if Life is Omnipotent and causes breath, again, why do we say man dies. Recently a famous movie screen star living, near here having been confined for life in a wheel chair died, doctors say, from an absence of will to live. This is a profound statement of universal truth. Jesus said: "My food is to do the will of Him who sent me that I may perfect His work" (John 4:34) and "If thou wilt enter into Life keep the commandments," To live Life abundant and everlasting, one has to have the will to Life by doing the commandments, or one dies the death for the desire or attraction to sin and all the consequent miseries and sufferings of existence in mortals. Old age and sickness are due to the mortal mind's misery hypnotized by attachment to sin, and its results seen everywhere in the world. With a true will to live by God's laws or commandments, and its practice, it is impossible to die the death, which is the reward for sin.

However, breath does give us all the cosmic energy to move and be animated. The explanation of this is given in Transcendental Truth Teachings XI on Pranic Force which accompanies this lesson but was written in the Andes in 1947 when I began to write on "Heliovora Living." Please read it now...

Having gained an explanation as to the cosmic ultraviolet energy being the force that Life uses for animation, rather than chemical reactions, carbohydrates, etc., of the "childish physical-chemical concepts," being the cause of motion, next we might look into whether food, or air gives substance for our body.

Reviewing the Scripture, it says: "There went a vapor from the earth, and watered the whole face of the earth, and the Lord God formed man of dust from the earth, breathing into his nostrils the breath of life, and man became a living soul." Whatsoever is possible once with God Law, is true always for He is immutable, and if man came from the dust and vapor that rose from the earth which was breathed by God or Life into man's organism to materialize or give substance to the soul of man, then this is the first natural law of our being. Books speak of Creation as a "beginning" which make it possible to grasp the Infinite concepts with the finite mind. But just because man measures the transitory nature of earth not what he calls time, this does not make this a true concept. Christ said, "I am the Beginning and the End," and with some study we see the first Creation of God is an Eternal Process and Principle. God's Law of Paradise is Eternal, in force always, to the end described in the Apocalyptic Celestial City of the Christ Kingdom. Man was a living soul thru the breath of Life in the Paradise of pleasures. The fruit he ate gave him pleasure, so he had the will or desire to live. Sinning by eating abominations, man lives in sorrow and suffering and loses the will to live very fast as shown when the early puberty and meat eating stimulated by eating seeds are taken up by man in Genesis, he gets a habit of liking the life span of around 100 years rather than near a 1,000 years potentiality of man in mortality after the fall even!

No matter if our food is the vapor and gaseous elements in the air, or the liquid and solids we eat which are to be assimilated, have to become gaseous vapors in the intestinal furnace, in all cases it is only the vaporized substances we build tissue from. In fact, the visible solid and liquid forms of food are poisonous in most cases. Proteins decompose to uric acid, the principle poison of auto-intoxication in the flesh. That nitrogen is assimilated from the air to combine with nascent hydrogen condensed in the intestinal tract, is a fact recognized by biochemists in which they explain that nitrogen gas builds tissues, is found in muscles and fibrous tissue, and is first of all the elements to leave a dead body starting tissue decomposition. And we have to say this to bridge the gap from understanding some kind of material as the carrier of Life, to materializing substance from energy. All substance is energy in the form of positive and negative electrical charges. Now the scientist Lakhovsky showed that organic growth and maintenance is the work of cosmic rays. He claimed the living organism is a materialization of cosmic rays, that they are a subtle stream of ultra electronic form and materialize into grosser minerals as they strike the earth's atmosphere so that the body is a materialization of "Cosmic Food." We see life with air as the only sustaining substance in some bacteria, and in some animals such as a turtle which lived nearly a century and a half in a cement foundation of a Visalia, California, building without food or water. But Lakhovsky proved air with its mineral elements not necessary by keeping unicellular organisms in a sealed test tube, and measuring the amount of iron they contained before and after a certain period of growth; found that the iron content of the cells increased as they multiplied, again showing living substance to be materialized from cosmic rays rather than being converted from other substances. In our "Heliovora" theory, another writer claims sunlight is converted into minerals in the body according to the spectral colors, each corresponding to different groups of minerals.

Metaphysics claims all visible things come from the invisible, just like ice and water is condensed from vapor in the air, and since science has proven all matter to be particles of electricity revolving in a certain intelligent order like the planets of the universe, one can see that the human materialization from the air is not a secret power of masters, but the common natural law we all live by. Moreover, the eating of heavy proteins creates an excess of uric acid that is claimed the cause of the body's degeneration and death by physicians, and yet as we explained in Lesson VI, proteins stimulate the reproductive powers (Life feeling the nearing to death in one organism seeks another) giving the illusory feeling of strength and well-being while the body ages and is eaten up.

Some research has been started divorced from the necessity of protein foods, but what about minerals to replace minerals in our cells, is a frequent question. However, let us take the examples of foods that contain iron such as spinach, chard, beets, etc. The iron they are so famous for is in the form of oxalic acid. But alas, oxalic acid is poison! This iron in food is boasted as curing so much iron deficiency disease, is in oxalic acid which poisons giving symptoms of oxaluria with highly pernicious consequences in distressing nervousness besides stones of kidney and bladder. It is claimed 20 times weight dissolved in water has power to cause death by acting on brain, spinal cord and heart, and cases of death from rhubarb are attributed to oxalic acid. Oxalic acid must leave the body unchanged like other mineral acids, because it cannot be oxidized in the body tissues. These facts are given in Dr. T. De la Torre's works.

Going thru the various natural health foods we find them all to contain some kind of poison, drugs or blood toxins, which of course, are effective in counter-acting other poisons we combine them within what we may call the "battle of poisons" to make us "live", or rather attempt to live life but destroy it too, by pleasures! If these poisonous substances are assimilated they would only poison us, and thus we see that we do not assimilate minerals, nor vegetable animal substances of a lower rate of vibration than human tissue. If we did we would become the same, turning into dead mineral deposits, vegetable cells or have bodies and flesh like that of cows and pigs. Yet we so get something from food which in vitamins is a certain frequency of radiant photo electrical ray energy, and in minerals it may be that each mineral carries spectral color vibration of sunlight that converts into this mineral potency (as indicated by Babbitt) though the mineral itself is not assimilated except as a poison, while in proteins it is definitely a pathological uric acid stimulation of the reproductive glands that gives us strength sensations.

In fact, eating destroys instead of supports Life! We do it for pleasure just like those who smoke, drink alcohol, and abuse their bodies in other ways and also live to be over 100 years of age just like those who are careful to avoid these habits, but this does not prove one could not live to be, 1000 years or more if a person avoided all false pleasure-seeking habits including eating and sex waste.

All this goes to prove that all our worldly knowledge or "science" is a hoax, motivated by the selfish financial gains of drug-peddling doctors, commercial scientists selling foods, drinks, smokes, and other habit-forming articles and gadgets to the slaves of "civilization." God in whose image man was made, was not to become a slave. This is man's price for self and sin. The idea of an individual free to sin as he pleases must be forsaken for God, our origin and end, and the Law we live by.

Now rather than attempting to prove foods are poisonous in detail, or how the invisible is the cause and origin of all visible forms in the everlasting process of Life Creation, facts on dozens of people who actually live completely on the spiritual plane without eating would be more convincing proof to upset all these secular "scientific" theories about life coming from the enjoyment of pleasurable foods. This formidable proof we give in the next lesson.

LESSON XVII

FAMOUS CASES OF CATHOLIC FOODLESS LIVING AND HOW CHRIST'S TRANSUBSTANTIATION FROM COMMU-

NION SUSTAINS SAINTS

The most convincing proof of Foodless Living and the fact that eating is not essential to Life but is a false pleasure-seeking habit, is the living truth of famous cases observed by millions of people already, and which anyone can have proof of in contemporary living mystics. So without using up any more of our limited space let us commence to condense information on the subject that there are volumes to be found in large public libraries if one interested. Your writer was first inspired about man living without food when a lad in high school in 1938, when he read some newspaper accounts (in our possession still) about the world-famous stigmatist of Konnersreuth, Bavaria, Therese Neumann, and also when this former self had no respect for religious people and least of all for Roman  Catholics. Living in the atmosphere of Americanism interpreted as freedom from being reminded of the consequences of sin in one's suffering and pleasures, anything to reform corruption certainly is welcome besides being examined constantly in suspicion and hate, in spite of the subjects good and even holy intentions. This is why hardly no one else hears about the living proofs of Christ's teachings such as the Catholic stigmatists except Catholics, and when they appear elsewhere the multitude of "Doubting Thomases" either search for a quick reason for denial or skeptically ignore occasion to know Christ and his story thru His wounds. Most so-called Christians prefer an oracle they search in the Old Testament Scriptures and somewhere in man's history of sins committed on earth he finds defense for his actions, believing because it is recorded that men warred on cities, killed all men, took women for slaves, confiscated all their wealth and lied and blasphemed God saying the Lord told them to do this in their records, man has the eternal right to sin and glorifies the freedom to do so.

After the Old Testament history along comes an ascetic denouncing the pleasures of the world, telling his disciples to forsake wives, parents and family, worldly possessions, lands and even be ready to give their very life for the Spiritual Government of God. This is all that was needed to make Jesus, God's Word of Love, the most hated man in his world. Today people still hate anybody or any Church that teaches asceticism or making statements such as Pope Pious XI in the Constitution "Umbratilem" saying the contemplative life is much more fruitful for the Church than the activity of teaching and preaching. Jesus gave his life for a true Christ for His Church, and there are people on earth who mock the idea that he died for our salvation. Listen if we never had a Jesus we would still be raising pigeons and turtles to sacrifice at the altar for our sins without the Gospel of Good News about the glorious way to salvation that proved successful in 19 centuries of great saints. To this day, Gandhi, and other non-violent pacifists are giving their lives rather than let world sin perpetuate itself thru them in lip-service or actions.

Now this oracle of the "letter that killeth" rather than quickens the Holy Life, has been perverted by those who fell from the original Catholic Church, because they hated the teachings of Christ, and they made their Bibles to their own liking, which caused the giving of cheap propaganda Bibles and the burning of fake Bibles by the Catholics. To illustrate how words were bent to the liking of the new translators, the Catholic Bible uses the words, "Do penance" for the kingdom of Heaven is at hand, but the Protestants mildly excuse themselves by merely saying one needs only repent. The Catholic footnotes explain the root words to mean "punishing past sins by fasting and such like any seller of goods or services, mildly says just, "Repent ye" and then they go on changing our Original Scriptures to give us a salvation thru only vicarious atonement saying all we got to do is believe in Christ and live happy in the word of sin because Jesus got our salvation for us without any need of effort on our part except joining a sectarian "saved" group. In Matt. 19:12 the Catholic footnote about "eunuchs" for the sake of God explains this as, "Continence practiced in view of the kingdom of God is better than married life" but the Protestants do not want others to interpret the Bible for them teaching sex is all right as long as you use contraceptives or get married and that continence is sin actually for neglecting one's duty in marriage.

Now unprejudice to Catholics in some slants such as oriental reincarnation which first Popes taught but now is anathema, the Roman Catholics do not reword things to a new meaning. And they do teach a re-incarnation of man or resurrection of the flesh while the Protestants ignore this, but talk of hell and heaven without the flesh which would mean no sensual body to suffer one's sins as we do now and always, and twist Mark 12:26 to say "touching the dead, that they rise" bringing in miracles where Jesus was only talking of the resurrection of the flesh as Catholics translate it. The Rheims version says in Mark 12:25 "they shall rise again from the dead," and "concerning the dead that they rise again," not only teaching that death is no victory over the flesh or escape from suffering for our sins in a body, but gives the reason why the first Church Fathers believed in the pre-existence of souls, speaking of our rising again and not just rising once when one dies. The Catholics have translated "the Orient on high hath visited us" explaining "the Orient" (eliminated from Protestant Bibles) as a title of the Messiahs giving evidence that His Light came from the East since His gospel and very words are found already centuries before in the teachings of Buddha and Oriental Avatars. But we can forgive the Protestants for these literal Bibles, because they started many on the road, who would have renounced any gospel they could not follow in the world with self-praise as to what "Christians" they were to the very letter of their Bible in their distinction of being "saved" thru an easy Bible.

As to Roman Catholics and the stories about them, what does it matter, their priests and people only profess the belief in the Apostles' Creed and Church doctrines and admit they don't have grace to live up to the teaching as their Saints often do. Is this any reason to "doctor up" our Bible and make a false teaching that is easier to follow, just because the Church and priests of the world can't be perfect, and to condemn those who teach the original discipline but have not the grace in this life to live up to it? "Wherein thou judgest another thou condemnest thyself of same thing."

But now to the living proof of the Apostles Creed, Stations of the Cross and other Church contemplations. How can one prove them. First by self-realization in Church and, second, observing the living gospel portrayed in living saints. After a millennium of darkness almost preceding Jesus and the First Christians, along came St. Francis of Assisi whom some have called the "Second Christ" who gave proof of Christ. Don't worry the worldly priests did not want much to do with him, spoke of him as a "heretic" because his Christ-like life embarrassed them and so it is with many saints of the Church. He possessed only one book, the New Testament (without the Jewish history of sin, the shield of sinners) and his simple life in nature loving all, calling the birds, fish, animals as well as man his brothers affirmed in his actions of eating no meat besides making Franciscans pacifists, and in poverty without worldly possessions that would make others envy him. St. Francis was the first stigmatist recorded in the history of the Church, which is a gift only achieved by those who give up own will and ideas of God and meditate on the true everlasting doctrine like the saints who know Christ Jesus to the extent of manifesting His wounds on their body. Now in our teaching on Yoga we show that Yogis obtain complete knowledge of anything by doing "Samadhi" or Supreme Rapture (Contemplation) on it. They identify themselves with the object so as to know its properties completely, and you see the record of these identifications of repeated contemplation on the bodies of Christian stigmatists. Stigmatists are only found in the Roman Catholic Church because they are the only ones that give the complete discipline that leads to the Intimate Union with God and Divine Rapture, while with other Christians, God-Union is merely an inexperienced belief. I would estimate there have been hundreds of stigmatists after St. Francis of Assisi, since Dr. Imbert Gourbegre counted only 321 in his book "La Stigmatization" (published in Paris 1894)

The artless soul, childlike character, love for birds, animals flowers found in St. Francis, today is again encountered in Therese Neumann, the great marvel of living demonstration of Christ in the Church of our century. The sight of her wounds bleeding as she contemplates Christ's Passion, her living without eating and other gifts have convinced Protestant leaders as well as Jews and even Masons of the 32nd degree to join the R.C. Church. In two years after World War II in 1947, 12,000 U.S. soldiers visited Therese in spite of her dislike of any exhibition or anyone photographing her. We have

given an elaborate description of Therese Neumann in Transcendental Truth Teachings VII, so we shall try to avoid details
given there. Therese was born on Good Friday, April 8, 1898
at Konnerareut, and please note that it is on holy days of the
Church (not astrological dates) that every great event of her
life took place. As a young girl she gave up dolls as soon as
she discovered they were not really alive, and she cared only
for biographies of Saints and books on religion, and refused to
bother with fairy stories, legends and fiction in her love of true
things. Came the first World War and she took over the men's
work, they being taken as soldiers, and she liked the plowing
and heavy work better than housework. There were a few
suitors interested but she refused them all for this pious girl
had planned her career as a nun for a mission in Africa, if God
willed! Then one day she was helping fight a fire, lifting water
buckets to a housetop and she dislocated her spine which
resulted in paralysis of the spine, blindness and sores yielding
an odor no one could stand in her room. Imagine the test of
these soul crushing experiences with which she was purified
for her "resurrection" to the Holy Life. From perfect health and
strength equal to men to not only a bed-ridden invalid but loss
of sight and abhorable degeneration. The paralysis took over
the throat muscles so she could not swallow, so she could
do absolutely nothing but fast and pray. She had taken the
"Little Flower," Therese of Lisieux as her spiritual helper and
on the day of her beatification, April 29, 1923, Miss Neumann
regained her sight to read even small print she had never read
before thru a miracle from devotion.

But the flesh was rotting away as fast as to make a
bone bare and she was advised to have the leg amputated.
The Next miracle in her continued fasting and prayer happened when Pope Pius XI canonized St. Therese of Liseiux on
May 17, 1925 which removed the dislocation of her spine and
healed the ulcers of her body, and on Sept. 30, 1925, the an-
niversary of St. Therese's death, Miss Neumann walked again
for the first time in seven years! This seven years Spiritual
Preparation for her holy mission was constant purgatory, and
in all the visits from her Saint she was instructed that "more
souls are saved by suffering than by eloquent discourses," but
in Lent season 1926 she also began taking the agony of Christ

upon herself, deeply absorbed in ecstatic vision of Jesus and His Crucifixion. And ever since this Lord's Passion on Good Friday, 1926, she has had the profuse bleeding of the nail wounds, wounds of hands and feet, the sword mark on the side and thorns in the head, every Friday, except after Christmas till Easter when the Church does not celebrate it. Long descriptions of what she sees watching Jesus start on His way to Calvary and later describes the alleys and houses along the route. The realism of her visions is shown also by the fact that when the crowning of thorns takes place she hears the words of derision in Aramaic, the common language in Palestine at the time of the Passion. She hears, "Salem, malka (je) hudaje! Salem, Mesicha! Salem, rebhutha! (Hail king of the Jews! Hail, Messiah! Hail Majesty!)." She speaks Aramaic as Jesus did 2000 years ago, not merely Hebrew, Latin, and Greek which certain "exposers" CLAIM COULD BE FROM HEARING PRIESTS CONVERSE, and yet this is a peasant girl of practically no education in her normal person. Think of the value of this clairvoyant vision on the facts beyond scriptural description in minute detail about Jesus, the truth seen from His life in eternity, rather than morbid phrases of books.

Now the relation between Foodless Living and Stigmatists is that although all ecstatics are not stigmatists, all stigmatists are ecstatics, and all Foodless Livers are ecstatics. The greatest technique of total abstinence among Christians is thru ecstasy after stigmatization, when all the sensual desires of the body are "crucified" for Christ. And most significant is that all stigmatists who are women (and out of 321 stigmatists only 41 were men) overcome menstruation thru fasting and prayer to gain their powers in Christian Ecstasy.

As we told you, Therese Neumann has taken no solid food since 1923 when starting a liquid diet of practically nothing but water and fruit juices to be followed by complete abstinence, neither eating nor drinking anything since Christmas 1926 except the tiniest particle of the Sacred Host in Church which disappears on the extended tongue outside of the mouth without being swallowed. Roman Catholic Bishop of Cleveland, Rt. Rev. J. Schrmevs tells us that Doctors in Universities of Berlin, Leipsic, Prague and Munich agreed that "deception and fraud are absolutely out of the question in the case of Therese Neumann." A strict Medical investigation of the case was conducted over a 15 day period, in which all water she washed in was measured, every move watched and yet losing weight when she bleeds in ecstasy, she gains six to eight pounds out of the thin air back to normal each time. Dr. Urban observed there was no "ausscheeidungen" (no excretions) of any kind which would result if food were taken.

Yet the yellow papers for instance the "American Weekly" Oct. 1939, have run articles saying she dried up dying of starvation, must have taken milk of something, and explain the stigmata observed by all as caused by hysteria.

However, the blood observed especially on the foot wounds does not drop directly to the bed she lies in according to gravity's pull, but flows upward to the toes, defying gravity, just as it trickled to the toes nearly 2000 years ago for Jesus on the cross vertically, which surely is nothing explainable as hysteria! Of course, M.D.'s are crying for more investigations, thinking this would be a fine "guinea pig"', but Herr Neumann knows there would never be any end if permitted and probably "heard of what they did to Louise Latiau" in such circumstances. Moreover, there is an insistence that it should not be Catholic doctors, but a "neutral clinic" because this is considered as a "Catholic" disease, which the "neutral" doctors want to cure with special "catholic" injections! I have an article from Babahoyo, Ecuador of March 8, 1952 telling of Miss Isabel Vergara who has the stigmatist bleeding every Friday, and of course, the paper says it should be an object of "investigaciones cientificas" but also the subject is believed suffering from attacks of hysteria! Especially is the phenomena of devotional God rapture disturbing to some because they, unlike common Oriental Samadhi ecstasy in which the contemplative becomes rigid losing signs of life to appear dead, result in "mimic" ecstasy (from the "Bhakta Yoga" technique of Catholic devotion), that is, they remain mobile and carry out definite movements.

This is explained: "A more than human power, be it God or an angel, acts upon, stimulates an inner organ which the Scholastics call the "sensus communis" (inward central sense). The same power carries the stimulus thru the fancy to outer sense organs. The speaker's inner idea is transformed by his fancy into outer sensory instruments and gestures." Besides Therese Neumann there was Maria von Moerl of Tyrol who was seen by 40,000 people between July and Sept. 1833 who were moved by her mimic ecstasy combined with visions of the Passion. Suppose a person became a mimic ecstatic in the midst of a city like Los Angeles or New York (and this is impossible as every breath of smog deadens brain cells), and began to have convulsions every Friday in which they grasped at imaginary thorns in the head, writhed with pain in the hands and feet that began to trickle blood from imaginary nail wounds and spoke in Aramaic! Our country with all its "religious freedom" has a special "interdenominational monastery" for all these, with "Catholic" besides interdenominational syringe dope injections that will create a synthesized artificial "purgatory" since none of our so-called mystics care to get the powers by years of doing extreme penance. Beware! Few, but there are some, who write me saying they are going to live without eating, and will do it just like that, besides being their own masters! Your writer visited hundreds of mystics and occult students in his travels of California, etc., and got some common information, most all had been to "an institution" and too many cases were so treated that they discouraged all spiritual development. Your writer was one who renounced human masters along with home, family, and wealth but fortunately the Supreme Master took him to remote Andies for his seven years of purgatory preparation to kill the old self in sin to make live the Christ Self. You still will have a master whether visible or invisible, and all cases one only gains the Supreme Treasure by crucifying self. As to an inspired individual path, this writer just fasted and meditated till he arrived at God-Rapture, but from there he was directed by the Cosmic Master to study and practice all the religious paths before he could synthesize a more effective and direct path for those he might try to aid to know the Supreme Goal. The Buddha claimed he was the product of 25 Buddhas before his Illumination giving the Path thru which he liberated thousands of souls to Nirvana later by mere compliance to the necessary rule for their case. The Theosophical Society is known for its interdenominational ideas, but this freedom only gives their group the greatest percentage going to mental institutions. Beware of powers with No price. Just writing "I am God" or chanting it in a strange tongue will not bring Permanent God ecstasy, though a disincarnate "Master" can get possession of you thus for strange thrills. Any power without penance still is paid later in suffering. So those living in any amount of population should put themselves into the care of a spiritual director (as most often one's immediate family first seek to "put one away") All over the U.S. a Catholic Priest (who have had more years in college preparation than any other profession, studying mysticism) can be found to make one ready for the convent, unless you are sure you have another master who knows the transition, or if stubborn about "no masters" go to a cave in the mountains where you are sure there will be no interference to your years of penance. "Grace" is not obtained, nor "Karma" paid, through doing one's own will but sacrificing it for the Will of God even in matters of penance. You want extreme favors, such as living without eating which demands pre-puberty retaining of the seed and ecstatic contemplation (to give you something to live for when sensual joys in eating are sacrificed), but no kind of Godhood comes except by the suffering Jesus, the Saints, the Buddha, and the Yogis had to go through. Are you better than all the Master Teachers, to be denied penance? Moreover, as M.D.'s show us percentage of cases of insanity sharply increase approaching the centers of cities, which is believed to be caused by the deadly effect of the poisonous air of our modern metropolises that deaden the brain cells. This explains why there is so much warning of the practice of Yoga by Westerners so often claimed to bring insanity, because breathing deeply of our cities' poisonous air not only eats and blackens the lungs to give respiratory ailments that follow the common cold, but deadening the brans cells the organism can't function rationally. To live on air, first get pure or genuine air, not deadly gases and smoke! We are herewithin endeavoring to demonstrate and teach you how to live without eating from personal experience and investigation, while the elementary health information on why ordinary people cannot live on air and newspaper reports on cases that do, are GIVEN BY: NATURAL SCIENCE SOCIETY, formerly of Orlando, Florida in writings of K. Klamonti. They have books available on this now.

Now let us contemplate the lives of some of these stigmatists who often were total abstainers of food, both of which powers may be attributed physiologically to their preservation of the youth vitality thru perpetuating the pre-puberty sex-conservation (without menses or pollutions) and spiritually thru ecstatic union intimately with God. The best known recent work on Therese is the "Story of Therese Neumann" by Albert Paul Schemberg from which I also quote the following:

"Louise Lateau lived all of her life (1850-1883) in her native village, Bois D'Haine, Belgium. At sixteen she nursed cholera victims in the parish when all others, even the members of their families, deserted them in terror. More than once she carried to the graveyard and buried them. At eighteen, Luise became an ecstatic and stigmatist, but continued to help support her poor family by sewing. An ecclesiastical board of inquiry and many physicians saw her in her agonizing Friday ecstasies of the sacred Passion and established the fact that for TWELVE YEARS her ONLY NOURISHMENT was weekly Holy Communion and three or four glasses of water each week. She never slept during this time, but spent the nights in prayer and contemplation while kneeling at the foot of her bed." "In a book dated 1947 we are told that when Louise Lateau became nineteen it became impossible for her to eat or drink anything on Fridays of her ecstasies. On other days, she was able to take small amounts nourishment, but with difficulty, and gradually all desire for food vanished. On March 30, 1871, Louise was able for the last time to take natural nourishment without suffering from the attempt. To please her troubled mother and in obedience to the command of her pastor, she tried to eat and subjected herself to this ordeal for some months. Finally it was admitted, reluctantly, that she needed no natural food, that all efforts to eat or drink caused her to suffer, and her complete abstinence did not detract the least from her health and cheerfulness."

The great St. Catherine of Siena is another stigmatist, who must have influenced other stigmatists under her name such as St. Catherine of Genoa, St. Catherine de Ricci and Anna Catherine Emmerich who came later, and who was able to make the wounds go away at times to escape attention thru humility and she also lived without eating. Other Catholic abstainers from eating were St. Lidwina of Schiedam, Blessed Angela of Foligno, Blessed Elizabeth de Rent, Dominic a Sazarri, etc.

Saint Nicolas von der Flue, the famed Swiss statesman called Buder Klaus, canonized May, 1947, whose home was Unterwalden, Switzerland, lived for 20 years without food or water, after renouncing his family and possessions. Therese Neumann is often asked to identify relics of saints, and being given one of Saint Nicolas von Flue she said, "Oh, my, that was a good man, for he loved the Saviour very much. And do you know, he ate nothing, just as I do. But he had it much better than I, for he was in the woods and the shining man (guardian angel) brought him our Lord (sacramented)." Some of these hermit saints received their "sacramental Jesus" at distances when not able to attend communion in body, the same as one should attend mass in spirit mentally if one's work does not permit one to go physically to the Church.

Here I would like to explain the mystery of why it is necessary to live celibate, not giving into marriage and moreover if one is married they have to forsake or renounce and hate (as the Bible says) one's partner in marriage besides other family relationships for God's Government to resurrect from the dead to the spiritual kingdom where we are to live without eating and enjoy bliss of the celestial life. You can imagine why people hated Jesus for exposing marriage and your writer is receiving a few protests from married students who "agree with all in Vitarianism except that they believe in the honor of marriage." This Teaching is not divorce with possibility of re-marriage, but absolute renunciation of the marriage relationship forever. This St. Nicolas von Flue abandoned his wife with ten children for the hermit's life in the Swiss mountains, just as many of our purest souls have given up family and the world no matter how immersed they were in it (the more difficult the renunciation the better it is for the soul) and the convents have saved many a pure sweet youth from intent of parents to sacrifice them to an ugly marriage slavery to get wealth. We keep repeating that anyone can become a virgin, wash away sins thru Christ, beginning this moment. There is no excuse in "Oh, I am married, I got three children the business needs me, etc." God and true longing for Him is Omnipotence, and if we pray even one whole night seeking hard enough, arrangements will be made available to have one's marriage partner live satisfactorily in one's absence, and willing friends, relatives or means, God reveals best who will care for the children if one cannot do it himself with present accumulations. Worse cases like that of St. Nicolas von Flue and other saints were solved, but the way comes only if one has the Will for God's way so that He can help you. If you renounce His way and aid, only the world will help you and deeper into worldly ways. Unless one makes haste in preparation, the chances for salvation in this supersonic world can be taken away too soon. "The Kingdom of Heaven is at hand," but now! No one lived without eating while married, this being a power manifest only in the original or restored virginity.

Jesus rebuked his mother at Cana saying, "Woman, what have I to do with you," showing we are to renounce all attachment created by the bestial form of reproduction, ignoring carnal relations for the Spiritual Brotherhood of all humans, and especially should man forsake living in sin with his wife because the love of marriage partners has been defiled by their first mutual sexual adulteration, forever a reminder of their lower love that led to sin as long as they have memory. This memory of sin is only eradicated by getting out of the old environment and relationships to live a new detached life of purity. Two people who have known the marriage act are constantly provoked by disincarnate elementals with reproductive desires, defiling one whether or not one physically or mentally accepts them by their mere presence, while the ascetic vow of restored virginity kills such desires giving one an emancipation from such obsessions. "Making love to a nun," etc., are phrases that illustrate the repulsion the worldly and earth-bound spirits have to the celibate vow, while even the strictest Catholic monastic life permits the nuns to receive Christ's Love sacramented from the priests unblemished in virginity. "I come not to bring you peace, but separation.....and a man's (spiritual) enemies shall be they of his own household." Renounce! And Jesus assured us reward for this forsaking of family in this present life and in Life Everlasting which is the Spiritual Love and Ecstasy. Nor does this forbid intimate association and undefiled love among the religious, just as the celibate Jesus accepted the love of woman, one who washed his feet, wiping them with her hair and kissed them, which to the amazement of others from his lauded beyond all their demonstration of love. Constantly he gave a touch of virtue or healing to others from his purity or creative powers. Sin needs bonds to check its growth as in marriage, but heaven is not bonds, limited or attachment, but Bliss and Life Unlimited. Marriage is necessary now in the world only because people eat the passion foods.

Furthermore it is only the touch of the celibate that can forgive sins, not just some "faithful" whose energies seed and leak in the sex, showing the wisdom of Roman Catholics forbidding marriage of priests. These "virgins" of the Church that consecrate their meditation on the Christ in the transubstantiation of the host to the body of Christ in the Holy Eucharist, thus give the host the priest's charge of Christ, the Man Immaculate, to unite with the feminine "Bride of Christ" creative force which gives the marvelous spiritual power of the sacraments Christ, the true "Vita" in creative balance on the spiritual plane. If you follow me here you will see how deluded some are by such acts as saving the "bread" (quarter sized piece of paper made of rice) showing it as "Christ Sacramented." The sacred host is like a holy vitamin, once discharging its super-solar energy to the body, it is dead again. Theresa Neumann and others know and can feel this energy in the host, being able to distinguish the Eucharistic Christ from an unconsecrated host. She sees a radiance with Jesus Christ in it when taking the host, supernatural symbolism being a wondrous Technicolor movie one sees in mimic ecstasy as some of us have experienced in communion, besides other Divine Rapture. This shows why some priests are holier than others for having prayed and fasted more and can give more of the Christ Virtue.

The fact that out of 321 having ecstatic identification in Christ Jesus in their bodies, ONLY 41 WERE MEN shows that the Eucharist consecrated by male celibates was not the complete factor to give other male celibates the power of abstinence from food. A contemporary to St. Francis and first Franciscans was another vegetarian, St. Dominic who founded the Order of Dominicans, who was visited by the Blessed Virgin and urged to propagate the Rosary as we now have it with its 150 "Hail Marys" and contemplation of the Joyful mysteries related to Immaculate Conception and the Glorious mysteries on the Ascension, Descent of Holy Spirit, Assumption of Mary into Heaven and her Coronation in Heaven, besides the Sorrowful mysteries of Christ's Passion Sacrifice. This added contemplation of Heaven thru the Ascension of the Glorified Master and the Holy Virgin, brought the Heavenly Life without eating and other blessings into the Church, and matches the Yoga contemplating of male breath "Pingala" and female breath "Ida" uniting to produce the "Kundalini Shakti" that ascends to "Samadhi" or God-Rapture with corresponding powers. It is the interchange, the union of immaculate male and female forces that sublimate our life into spiritual force and life. The Roman Catholic Church's holy pictures contemplate the sisters kneeling, receiving the blessings of the master Jesus and the brothers on knees before the Heavenly Queen which we see is a necessary intercession for the powers of balanced transmutation.

In paragraph 15 of "Lessons from the Life of Love-Wisdom" I tell you of my first relationship with the Virgin, no girl in school ever came up to the immaculate beauty of the "dream girl" within, and all seemed depleted of this touch of virtue at high school age, while I did and do like to entertain little girls of innocence not defiled by menstruation or lewd relations, of early school age. A little girl's mere smile has often radiated strength in moral morale for the day's hard work. In Quito on Sundays I used to enjoy hiking out in the country with students carrying their little girls who couldn't endure the distance on my shoulder "como el elfante." In rare occasions when people try to drag me away to an evening's pastime, they find me a sad entertainer, except in cases where disciples let me display my ego in spiritual lecturing. Like a child, I feel like bursting out crying unless I can be alone in peace with my Celestial Lover which I think justifies my early retiring with coming of darkness with the rest of nature though I sleep about three hours only. A "date with the Virgin," the Mother of God in all, mightily, spiritually gives rebirth of our Christ, Whose Light can illuminate to us with the Profounder Truth. Giving up the passion foods that materially stimulate one's lower sex force in the Vitarian Diet, we gradually prepare you for the super-natural or spiritual source of power so the body can live on the spiritual plane on spiritual food thru balanced sublimation. In meditation I find the Spiritual Virgin, not of the physical plane nor of the astral (or mental, etc.) plane, but of the third world or Celestial Plane, coincide in body position to my body, identifying consciousness of a balanced Father-Mother God in union to liberate one from the Three Worlds to the Absolute or Omniscience, though in the lower preparatory aspects the feeling of full breasts and other female intricacies only rudimentarily developed in man, invigorate the body in regeneration and vitalize the mind with resolution and resourcefulness in the conquest of supernatural ideals. Transcendent Wisdom came thru the bisexual, but virginal, Love Rapture, divorcing the soul interests and body from subjection to so called world realities for the Bliss of Cosmic Truth.

You may have never studied the devotion to the Mother of God and incomprehensive position of Christ as Son of God, or vice versa in the mysteries of the Rosary and the Eucharist (which were not meant for material-reasoning minds) but here is being celebrated every moment of the day somewhere on earth this Super-conceptual Love, and you may not dare be seen in a Catholic Church by friends, yet here are spiritual things we experience even before studying Christian Mysticism living a moral, natural life telepathically entering the Holy Spirit of the Church. Hindu Yogis have their "Inner Woman" so as to have no use for touching an outer woman. Tantric Yogis and Taoist Masters achieve extreme longevity and foodless living thru a celibate associating with young virgins. When the women in bondage to control sin will be shameful if not unknown, all capable of a resurrected in-the-flesh knowledge of virginal love rapture without sin, living saints taking the place of crucifixes and Virgin portraiture. Next lesson we shall continue with  more cases of foodless living, comparing preparatory methods of Yoga, etc., developing our synthesis of all forms of religious rapture into Vitarian Virginal Spiritual Sublimating Ecstasies for the Direct Path to Spiritual Identification with Wisdom and Bliss.

LESSON XVIII

PRACTICAL WAY OF SPIRITUAL ATTAINMENT SOLVES FIRST PROBLEMS OF EXISTENCE FIRST, MORE NON-EATING CASES, REPRODUCTIVE TUMORS

In the Vitarian Way, for the first time in the history of religions, philosophies and sciences, you are now given a practical way of spiritual living to give one the experience of knowing the Transcendent Truth, which is Blissful Peace and Eternal Serenity. Never has the root cause of world suffering been found, this being always by-passed even by the great sages in teachings and even if taught it was not eliminated in practice.

Jesus Christ could only vaguely start to tell men of his day what this was not finally. He had to bid men farewell saying they were not able to bear the teachings He had to give, and that the Spirit of truth would come to reveal it. (John 16:12.

The ancient Yogis taught that by conquering desires we can gain Liberation and they tried to undo past errors by inflicting injury to the body, mortification to cancel Karma. The Buddha, Siddhartha Gautama, with the gospel of moderation, "the Middle Path," indicated the way of the Emancipating Truth in a more principled renunciation, discerning and living the Law. Buddha said the whole world had its origin in lust, that is, the procreating desire is the basis of all creations, and the attainment of Immortality was in the destruction of birth (action, desires, etc.) which will make suffering and death cease as the result or effect. Siddhartha, the Buddha, was able to give out the deepest abstract transcendence in "Wisdom, but when he spoke saying, "Giving away our food we get more strength, giving away our clothes we get more beauty, founding religious retreats we reap the perfect fruit of the best charity" he found a strong opposition from the world. The penance of the humiliating advocacy of nakedness and fasting, giving up one's food and clothing or the first necessities of our world life, naturally is most opposed by those who want to appear religious and yet enjoy the pleasures of the body. So when some of the nuns and monks took to the woods without clothes and to half starve, there was overwhelming opposition.

And even the Buddha had by-passed the first essentials in giving up the material life for the spiritual. He went out to live alone in the forest seven years in penance, fasting except for one hemp seed a day, the combination of extremes to neutralize his good purpose. He found that with these years of penance he did not extinguish desire and acquire ecstatic contemplation, but had weakened his body so he could not care for himself nor was he even able to think coherently anymore. The traditional story then tells us that he met a maiden who made religious offering giving him food, so that he regained strength and entered his famous Ecstatic Bodhi Contemplations of Truth. The observing ascetics first thought the encounter with the maiden as evil, slipping of his religious zeal, and rather than recognize the influence of the balancing of spiritual forces between virgins of opposing sexes giving a release to the liberating power, even the Buddha said it was the food, from which he reasoned the gospel of moderation in food, not feasting nor fasting completely as necessary for spiritual conquests. Thus he forbade his disciples to use raw seeds as he had done in his seven year forest penance (besides meat), which ruined his efforts, because the substance taken in such small quantities congests in the intestines, poisoning the body by stored accumulation, and worse seeds as he used give passionate desire that even seven years of only a seed a day could not cure. Ever since man began to eat, he has believed food was necessary and his whole life is built on than idea! If the Buddha had washed out the intestines with water and fruit juices for seven years, he would then have been able to live plump in face and limbs without eating as do the modern total abstainers. He was quite right that such penances, whether it be the commonly ridiculed act of holding one arm in the air constant till it withers, or such imprudent methods of near fast ing that withered his body to skin and bones, have no spiritual value, though they are paying up a little past Karma instead of plunging deeper into sin. And so Buddha and his disciples preached the gospel of Emancipation "Nirvana", yet slaves to food depending on the laboring men, and not planting anything because it prepared births to reap the fruits of such acts and cultivation killed worms in the earth.

This contradiction in the principles of religious living has the western "practical thinkers" indignant. Modern India's famines and other problems are blamed on the hordes of beggars who teach giving up all worldly pursuits, yet depend on the world to exist. But worse, woman is made the scapegoat of all the troubles of man, which not only is the suggestion indicated in Buddha's teachings and Yoga literature of the orient, but also in the Christian religious life thru the past centuries, manifesting even in such sacred grounds as the Trappist monastery needing a sign at the entrance prohibiting women on the premises, again debasing women as the cause of Passion and evil. However, what can be expected from human bodies nourished on reproductive substance, and slaughtered carcasses even, except that very same quality they crave in food and are not able to forsake? Procreative and flesh foods build passionate carnal man.

Moses, beside other ancient religious founders, recorded the legendary first man and the first commandment given to man. This commandment had to do with the most important thing, the great factor in life of man which is the basis of all his endeavors, that is, food. The original sin was thru eating, and all other sins followed from it. When God was forsaken as the complete endeavor in man's life to earn bread, suffering and sorrow was the fruitage of his separation.

No one in the world wants to hear this! Man of all times says, "I would rather die than fast!" Nor are we going to use better psychology to help anyone overcome this prejudice. Our doctrine is ridiculous to the world, but the Truth it is, and if understood it would eliminate the world of ego-centric illusion.

Now speaking to any religious person of most any denomination and stating that food has anything to do with one's spiritual life, the quick retort is that Jesus said, "Not that which goeth into the mouth defileth a man, but what cometh out of the mouth, this defileth a man." This is, however, a most impractical observation. Take poison, or go on a spree of liquor and heavy foods and see if you don't get sick and curse or hate everything around you, if not die. Observe the paragraphs before this (St. Mark 7:3-23) and one sees this only referred to washing one's hands, dishes and pots before eating. However, if we would advocate the hermit's kitchen habits I am sure it would find ourselves labelled "not hygienic", not "teaching the doctrines and precepts of men" that Jesus therein denied. Germs won't hurt you, is the truth he spoke herein. He says, to eat with unwashed hands and special kitchen hygiene, "entereth not into the heart but goeth into the belly, and goeth out into the privy, purging all meats." Whether hygienically handled or not, matters little if the food is the result of killing to feed on a fast-decomposing carcass or taken to stimulate the procreative desire, which in the blood "out of the heart proceed as evil thoughts, adulteries, fornications, killing, thefts, covetousness, wickedness, deceit, blasphemy, pride and foolishness."

But notice that Jesus acknowledges the fact that food is eaten to push out the decomposing waste in the intestines, purging the body of wastes, rather than for need as a nourishment. And to definitely confirm the fact that food can affect the heart and soul, He said, "Take heed to yourselves lest perhaps your hearts be overcharged with surfeiting and drunkenness and cares of this life," tying in what we said above as to eating, original sin and suffering from such life pursuits. "SEEK NOT WHAT YOU SHALL EAT or what you shall drink," for those who really seek and believe in Christ do not hunger for material foods nor drinks.

But just like the Orientals the western religionists have sought a different interpretation to the simple plain obvious meaning of the Genesis First Commandment. Anything to be true in a parable or as a symbol needs to have literal truth also, but man would rather avoid this fact, saying that eating the forbidden food really means partaking of sex as the original sin, because secret eating practices are not possible, food needing a system of production, but sex can be secret, and even if it is blamed as the original sin, the sinning hypocrites subconsciously schemes that in this hiding he could still appear a man of virtue for merely saying this sex abuse is sin thus referred to in the First Law given unto man in Paradise.

So men go on feeding passion with passion producing food and fighting sin by resolutions to repress it. Lust was not first, but the symptom of the Cause of Suffering, the sin being in man eating forbidden food. Adulterating or defiling the body with seeds and animal substance sends lasciviousness, fornication, murder to the heart.

It is not necessary to take for granted any Bible legend about the first man. An eternal Genesis is in man forever. Some of you know from experience, in perhaps the first knowledge of the opposite sex you had in pre-puberty childhood secretly playing games in which the curious little ones excite each other in turn by manipulation to enjoy a minor ecstasy which in children before puberty is fully enjoyed without any loss of seed. This in youth, but from the ages of 10 years to 14 years the degenerative effects of passion stimulating foods set in, and the body begins to lose the seed.

Notice that with wrong diet, later in Genesis, the age of the beginning of puberty or child bearing, and the longevity of man decreased astoundingly. At first the sons of God had the longevity potentiality of nearly a thousand years, and reached puberty bearing children only after about a century of life, but when "the sons of God saw the daughters of men that they were fair, and they took them wives of all which they chose." so that having children already in the twenties, man is only given a life span of 120 years by the Creator. And with the increase of wickedness, God, the Universal Law, destroyed this man from earth in the Flood, but think of the present world sin ever on the increase, how can it survive? Jesus said we should be like little children to receive the Celestial Kingdom when explaining about what adultery is, because like man first created in God's image mentioned in Genesis, children do not have shame in sex, preferring to be naked rather than clothed, nor can they be de-filed in the loss of their seed. This again confirms the gospel in "whosoever is born of God, committeth not sin, for his seed abideth in him and he cannot sin," as man is in his pre-puberty stage of eternal Genesis known in childhood.

Now for the benefit of the Bible skeptics, let us compare the reports from the more unprejudiced medical research given in "The Ideal Sex Life" that records the findings of Johannes Rutgers, M.D., famed Dutch birth control advocate (whose methods we do not approve, however), which gives the painstaken observations in the field of sex. Medical research found that before puberty or before a child is conscious of sex because of reproductive development functions, children have erections from reasons yet unexplained by science, though our system of education based on the adult viewpoint teaches children to suppress sexual tumefaction as evil. Now in spite of the evidence that tumefaction is not from any reproductive desire or lust, occurring before any possible seed propagation, we are supposed to suppress it, and yet suppressing this most vital function of the prostate in man and clitoris in woman, we have robbed the human race of an essential part of its regenerative system. Because of human superstition and tradition, man and women have become half sexes of rudimentary development in these creative centers, and so also the brain is only fractionally evolved, the lungs are only partially used to get solar force when they should sustain man with a breath of life and throughout man seems atrophied from the legendary giant God created him in powers if not physique. Medical studies have comprehensively analyzed the generative organs, the progress of procreation, etc., but admit that in all their investigations they paid no attention to the regenerative system, do not know the function of the prostate, clitoris and have only started studying the glands of the region suspected to secrete rejuvenating hormones. Yoga calling itself the Eternal Science and of Immortality, in ancient teachings claims this the fountain of youth and the basic center of spiritual power, ecstasy and creation of spiritual being, but does so cautiously perhaps having lost the infallible keys to the Celestial Kingdom. The Yogi observes the two currents of energy, solar-male and lunar-female, unite at this basic center to form the ascending spiritual power that transforms man from the physical to a spiritual being of power and a fountain of bliss. The medical men note that the prostate (clitoris in women ) is a specialized organ for the climax of blood pressure, because it has two arteries to carry the blood there but has only one vein to bring the blood back to the heart from there, -so that with the two arteries (male and female currents) and the ascending prostate-to-heart vein that is increased to new life, we have the Yoga system of the body energy currents described from secular science. This creates the second-heart action in increased circulation for prostate activity giving elation of rejuvenescence (along with hormone activity thus induced) besides concentrating and transforming the body's opposing energies into one spiritual force, rapture that awakens powers to finally liberate man in illumination.

Again it is observed by medical men that only man with his immense brain power (and soul sensitivity) has tumefaction, the regenerative action, distinguishing him from the mortal beasts and enabling him to attain superior powers. The student of Yoga is instructed to sit on one heel and vibrate the body thus stimulating prostate activity in Siddha Asana used to awaken spiritual powers "by forcing the Kundalini Serpent out of its cave of hiding" in this region. It is noted by the medics that the mechanics of erection prevent the flow of semen in fullest degree, even cutting off passage, except when the thrill of waste if often, making the organs sluggish, showing prostate activity as regenerative rather than for sex waste. Dr. Rutgers observes that no drug can take the blood away from the brain, the opposite pole of the body, speculating that erection could thus be valuable in the bursting of blood vessels in the brain due to brittleness from arteriosclerosis in attacks of paralysis and apoplexy, and pities those having lost the "regulator of the body's blood circulation thru impotence."

Outstandingly shocking to some may be to know that reproductive cell production is tumour-shedding, which can develop into serious pathological results observed in the abuse of sex and age. Not only is menstruation abortion, as we quoted from other medical sources in Lesson 113, but the formation of reproductive tumors we call germinal cells or sexual fluid shows the setting in of the process of degeneration in which the Life Essence of the body seeks to perpetuate various bodies to carry on since the original one has been corrupted in sin with wages of death rather than capable of Life Everlasting. These research men seem to be agreed that reproduction originally was bisexual or hermaphroditic but has degenerated thru the influence of civilized life. Dr. Rutgers claims sex stimulation is due to the "consumption of spicy food and other stimulants, especially alcohol, all superfluous nourishment, especially of an albuminous nature" besides meat eating in man's diet. "Biologically considered, any kind of tissue formation, even of a pathological nature, is the expression of a certain growth energy which must be present to produce the tissue formation at all"....."when the reproductive cells have once become separate from the parent cells they must be discharged from the body"...."The essential constituent of the seminal fluid is the microscopic sperm cells, harvest of an embryonic tumor"...."Even in regards to this discharge, the reproductive cells occupy a position intermediate between the increase of growth on the one hand and the tumors of age on the other hand."..."As relief is always experienced after voiding of pus, so sexually, desire is relieved every time the reproductive cells are cast forth."..."In pathological tissue formation, however, the surgeon's knife is nearly always required to remove the tumor." And after these phrases we quote from Dr. Rutgers, he goes on to discuss the pathological nature of childbirth needing surgical assistance, all of which seems to be an evolution of good to him, but is not natural or spiritual to us. Instead of the viewpoint of sin, or pathological sexual reproduction and abuse as the chief and normal function of the sexual organs, if we looked for the wholesome function of spiritual power and bliss herewithin, more could be accomplished for man's salvation. The Vitarian philosophy looks on vegetable albumins; seeds including nuts, grains, legumes, etc.,-as superfluous protein that only convert into irritating toxins that inflame the regenerative centers to produce the tumorous growth of generative cells on the "mother cells" in the ovaries and testes, since some of us not eating vegetable proteins for years have the direct assimilation of all necessary nitrogen from the atmosphere. This parasitic tumorous growth of reproductive cells in seed-eating vegetarians and nut-eating fruitarians, -saping the vitality of youth, giving body wear-out, age and inability to attain the state of foodless living, we believe is the pathological degeneration first known to man in the original genesis as well as the genesis of any person in childhood, while the even more poisonous conversions from animal proteins of lacto ovo vegetarian and meat diets is believed by many physicians to give the irritating toxins that eat the live tissue in chronic tumors, cancers and other tissue inflammations characterizing most disease. Loss of seed is sin, and the Eternal Youth Life comes thru regaining the pre-puberty power of the incorruptibility of the flesh, thru fasting and prayer to restore man's power over death that came eating the forbidden food of Paradise.

The Buddha prophesied upon letting women take up the Holy Life, "If women had not received permission to go out from the household life, and enter the homeless state then would the pure religion have lasted long, the good law would have stood fast for thousands of years. But since women now have received the permission , the pure religion will not now last long, the good law will now stand for 500 years." Here is the admission that he had not fathomed the relation between woman, sin and lust. He did not know how to make himself pure as a little child to be incapable of losing seed or lascivious thoughts except by eliminating women. Yet he and his disciples fearing sin and women, unconsciously were drawn to them for no one else could they beg food from. Had they emancipated themselves they would have not needed food from worldly labor. However, not needing food, they would have not lost seed to sin, and even the exhilarating association would not have been so condemned but sanctioned.

Now true to Gautama Buddha's statement, 500 years later came another Enlightened One, a Buddha, now called the Christ in the West, who condemned not women, but instead healed them of their issue giving them the teaching of fasting and prayer, commanding the baptizing (of the body

inside and outside) with water and Holy Spirit for the remission
of sins! Just as Gautama was conferred his 49 day ecstatic
Bodhi contemplation of Truth to become the Buddha or Enlightened one after the interchange of spiritual force from the
maiden who fed him, just as in the last lesson we described
the Saints of the Church received a virgin interchange of
complementary balancing spiritual force in holy Communion
for ecstatic God Union and foodless sustenance and stated
as a generality that Transcendent Wisdom came thru bisexual
virgin Love Rapture,-Jesus became the Christ in its meaning "Anointed One" in our sacred history recording when the
woman anointed his body for the Great Sacrifice. In Mary's
Love for Him demonstrated by washing and kissing his feet
and anointing His body with costly essences, in envy they
ridiculed Him for permitting it, but He crowned this woman's
love above all the others and commanded this act to be taught
saying, "Amen, I say to you, wheresoever this gospel shall be
preached in the whole world, that also which she hath done
shall be told for a memorial of her." Jesus exemplified what
later became the sacraments of the Church, that is, John ad-
ministered Baptism of Jesus before He took up the Penance of
40 days of fasting, Peter confirmed Jesus as The Christ, Son
of God, and the Apostles partook of his Holy Eucharist, but it
was the beloved Mary Magdalene that had the higher sacraments in Extreme Unction when she anointed his body for the
burial and Holy Orders when she was the first to receive him
after the resurrection in the Heavenly Ascension. Christ thus
restored the equal spiritual status of women and men, if not
directing women to a part in "priesthood" if virginity is restored
as in the healing of Mary's issue and cancellation of sins,
though up to now the Church is directed by a male priesthood,
prejudice to women. Ancient woman was considered with
attributes eligible to become a priestess, but when man began
to war, woman became slave of conquest who had to live with
him, bear his name, be his property and so it was instituted as
marriage and men priests in religion, but the future perfection
lies in the original equality of both as known in Paradise and
as Gal. 3:28 explains Christ as neither male nor female. All this
points to an interdependence of male and female for spiritual
sublimation in God's Government. Jesus instituted Holy communion saying we take of the fruit of the vine in commemora-

tion of him yet when Martha criticized her sister Mary for sitting in communion "to hear his word rather than help her serve," Jesus justified Mary in giving no importance of food and such things and to regard the spiritual.

Presenting some of my new conceptions relating to the Holy Virgin and bisexual sublimation of solar energies to the raw-foodist Roman Catholic Priest, Dr. Navas of Quito, Ecuador, who is head of "Integral Naturism" and Kneipp movement there, I was answered by his letter saying, "I also honor the Virgin clothed in the Sun and she constitutes a necessary complement so I do not become hardened with isolation charged only with masculine electricity," and complementing all my on completer naturism and "Heliovora" sustenance form sunlight when I lived in Lake Quilotoa in 1947. However, he suffered as did St. Francis of Assisi from persecution from his immediate superiors who tried to forbid his naturism and eating of only raw foods, but like St. Francis sought audience from the Pope who understandingly accepted him, so also Dr. Navas told me the Archbishop in Quito learning his troubles had said, "If I had my life to live over again, I would do just as you are doing!" Truth will spontaneously conquer world ignorance, though at first as Jesus admitted, in this world blessings will bear persecution.

Now let us study some more of the both practical and spiritually sublime examples of Foodless Living on the Heavenly Plane of life. We have mentioned Yogis living in the Himalayan snows, which sounds most fantastic, but recently in the reports on the climbing of Mt. Everest, we are told of enormous footprints in the snow at 25,000 food elevations which the people there attribute to snow dwellers, "snow men", but the Swiss climbers could only guess as belonging to enormous apes. That men can be enormous we have proven by human skeletons near 22 feet tall I mentioned found in the high Andies, and that such men could adapt to snow let us tell you of a case here in the U.S. The Associated Press in Spokane, Wash., recently wrote; "Willis Roy Wiley is a husky, healthy, 68 years old specimen of manhood who for 32 years has been practicing the theory that the proper attire for Northern Winters is a pair of shorts and a heavy beard. He gradually removed the gar-

ments of civilization until he was wearing only shorts. His body
became so accustomed to life in the raw that now he says
he is no more bothered by weather than any other unclothed
animal. The severest winters when the temperatures drop
to 30 below, find him wearing only his khaki shorts and in 32
years he hasn't even had a case of sniffles. Dr. Arthur Lien,
head of Spokane County Health Dept. says Willie's skin has
become leathery and board tough. "Thirty-two years of rugged
living has developed a layer of insulation fat which increases
his weather tolerance." About the same time early this year
(1953) I was sent a clipping saying Wonder girl, "17 year old
Dhanalakshmi, has been living without food or water since the
end of May 1952. Completely baffling the medical world, she
is healthy and pursues all normal activities. She actually lost
weight when forced to take food." Thus evidence of attributes
of the snow dwellers in the super-altitudes of our planet is to
be found in the world visible to all, from people we describe as
living without food or drink, (it would not need be only enormous apes have this super-human power to live in the snow
without food) and from excavations there is evidence of humans being giants in the Past as also mentioned in Genesis,
so why not now. Naturists have adopted to cold weather, sleep
in snow surroundings, nude, except for a sheet and our study
of the organs only rudimentarily developed in man, we find
that large breasts in women do not mean more milk outside
of pregnancy, or lasciviousness, but among functions in original hermaphroditic humans this was for a graceful design to
distribute the fat lobules over the lungs, heart, etc., in protection from cold atmospheres, etc., capable of tumefaction to
increase and warm the circulation besides a spiritual warmth
characteristic in women, unlike the ugly folds seen in the over-
fat persons.

Certainly the best known description of a Yogi living without eating is given in Paramahansa Yogananda's book "Autobiography of a Yogi." He describes, "Giri Bala the great woman Yogi, who has not taken food or drink since 1880," and whose "non-eating state has been rigorously investigated by the Maharaja of Burdwan." Yogananda is also pictured with her in a Photo taken in 1936 at her home in the isolated Bengal village of Biur. The story goes that when she was a child she had an insatiable appetite, for which her parents scolded her mercilessly. One day when about 12 years old after such an occurrence she stated "I shall never touch food again as long as I live," which was only answered by a retort, "So, how can you live without eating, when you cannot live without overeating?" Then she sought a Master who after a Vedic ceremony "initiated me into a Kria technique which frees the body from dependence on the gross food of mortals. The technique includes the use of a certain mantra and breathing exercise more difficult than the average person could perform." When Yogananda asked to be taught the secret, she answered, "I was strictly commanded by my guru not to divulge the secret. It is not his wish to tamper with God's drama of creation. The farmers would not thank me if I taught many people to live without eating! It appears that misery, starvation and disease are whips of our karma which ultimately drive us to seek the true meaning of life," and as to the purpose of her being singled out to live without food she said, "To prove that man is Spirit. To demonstrate that by divine advancement he can gradually learn to live by the Eternal Light and not by food." Other facts about Srimata Bala are that she can control her heart and breathing, has contemplative vision of great souls, sleeps very little, has no bodily excretions, and the Government head conducted investigations, having her locked up for 2 months at a time in a room at his palace to prove her non-eating state.

A similar case was given in "India's Message" (Jan. 1932), which states; "Giribala Dassi, sister of Baba Lamboxar Dey, a practicing pleader of Purulia, has been living for the last forty years without taking any food, not even water, and has been doing her regular household duties with no apparent injury to her health. Many respectable persons can testify to the truth of this statement."

Now the Yogis say as did Giri Bala, the technique or "Kria" is mainly in mantra and breathing more difficult than the average person could perform. Yogis spend many years if not a lifetime doing extremely difficult postures and breathing, besides other complications unadaptable to the Western body and mind, expending a great amount of effort, while the Christian contemplatives get it spontaneously without the physical effort and unnatural methods, though both depend on ecstatic sublimation of the baser sex energies. This shows an overlapping, that is, it is not a special ritual or special exercise, but the contemplative sex sublimation that does it, though the elements of breath control and holy meditation act spontaneously in the opposite cases. Yet the Christian saints of total abstinence and ordinary Yogis who don't eat, age and die about the same as ordinary people. However, Tantric Yogis and Taoist Masters have done all three in their technique of sex sublimation by charging their bodies through the balancing interchange of forces sleeping together chastely with young virgins, to achieve what they call "air-eating," besides conquering age and realizing longevity in cases up to 800 years. But this Tantric Technique is also the most dangerous besides efficient method, which in turn has corrupted the greater percentage of religious, priests, and priestesses to mere prostitution in temptation aroused thru careless observance of the practices. Too much caution can never be given about sex fire, which without a master or mature understanding can deplete one to lowest immorality, disease and insanity. This also classifies the modern medical teaching of "ideal sex life in marriage." In the Tantric Technique the results are not permanent with only 2 or 3 years duration in food abstinence usually since the power of ecstatic interchange is lost thru familiarization just as worldly love fades fast. Immediate constant contact of a magnet to objects neutralizes the magnetism in a short time, while using them for magnetism at intervals conserves their power indefinitely.

And using an induction coil to make an electromagnet we can control the attracting forces, that is taking in a Higher Potentiality, than the one inherent in the ordinary magnet or man, we can sustain an Eternal (Love) Potency besides control the inherent human power over depletion in the marvelous human electromagnetic mechanism. If not of the same mental powers, constant contact and in unconscious state of sleeping can be used as a black art to sap the vitality of youth, and generally sleeping together is not a spiritual communion as when two people meet in interchange of both love and wisdom as is told of Jesus and Mary in occasions, before He stilled the sea in a storm, when Martha objected, the anointment for His burial, etc. God Contemplation should be the motive and goal in virginal sublimation, not the power of non-eating nor pleasure in the way.

For these reasons we have presented a profounder synthesis to perfect the natural Vitarian Technique for Foodless Living, since the efforts of the past have produced only a few results, and are not sage, efficient or practical for the average person to try. It is too much left to chance, none of the systems having a transition bridge in which the incorruptible state of the body begins to manifest while one is still eating and then spontaneously leaves off eating without superhuman sufferings or dangers. Instead of a cure for menstruation, Hindu Yoga profanes woman, forbidding her from going to the temple, at times, and forbids a Yogi even to look at her, for even the yogi though eliminating losses, is not passion-free, having to eliminate women instead. The Tantric and Taoist goes to the other extreme, courting danger in woman, eliminating holiness from the temple, degrading religion to prostitution, etc., as is criticized of the Central Asia cults. In the west the Church shows ruthless abstinences, and women are only favored in abstinence from food thru interchange with priests, except in denominations completely neutralizing interchange from sublimation, by marriage. The cessation of menstruation or "amenorrhea" and kinds of impotency in males are classified diseases resulting from anemia, worry, emotional unbalance, diabetes, kidney disease, tobacco, blood acidity, rich protein diet, psychological repression, etc., by medical authorities. Sainthood, ecstatic sustenance and longevity are not proved by pathological conditions, and eventually age will give most all the cessation of losses in spite of a sustained passion. In contrast to this ordinary type of celibacy, Vitarianism holds that the incorruptibility of the flesh requires cognizing that the fountain of youth is not in the fluids produced to shed the reproductive tumors, but is in the rejuvenescence system of the prostate (clitoris), hormone secretions, etc., which become the second heart for body, mind and soul transmutation. Only can we hope to return to a Heliovora life if we return to the complete bisexual function of all our organs, some of which are only rudimentarily developed in the half-integral male or female, and this can come by sustaining psychic-stimulation from both sexes, of all organs, as was found in the original perfect God-created hermaphroditic race.

There are a number of other cases of living without eating, and of special mention are those we obtained thru exchange of information with Natural Science Society, formerly of 2803, Bumbay Street, Orlando Florida. Your writer has avoided city atmosphere as a poison as bad as using cigarettes, alcohol, meat, toxic foods, etc., so I forget to mention this worst enemy of "naturists", hygienists, vegetarians, healthmen, but Kenyon Klamonti of this Society shows how the city air intensely and constantly poisons man and vegetation around cities, while the other poisons are taken occasionally. We have a clipping from Frankfurt, Germany on Willy Schmitz who recently fasted taking nothing but water and cigarettes for 79 days sealed in a glass cage. Klamonti tells of Oswald Beard, wounded in World War I in the stomach, who for ten years has taken nothing more substantial than tea spiked with cream and sugar, about 60 cups a day which dietetics would claim inadequate,- which only points out the "Nutritional Myth." Listening to reports of people living over a hundred, most are described to eat meat and often drink alcoholic drink, while teetotalers and vegetarians with an unjust indignation do not show up better. However, in the following examples of noneating we cannot find confirmation of any reliable investigation other than newspaper reports given, which we have found to print anything for sensation and are built of the imaginings of some reporters, often. The Catholic abstainers mentioned in preceding lesson have been the target of investigation of the whole world with a great deal of literature to found on them and the Church seeks accuracy of description for the benefit of future seekers. The cases such as Giri Bala are reliably studied in Yoga also. Even more skeptical than news reports would we classify the hidden "Occult" knowledge which affirms some Count St. Germain, some master, etc., lives without food. Years ago when first arriving in Los Angeles, Calif. I found a number of Occult students carrying rumors that a blonde American Yogi, who was a cook in a big hotel there, lived on the vapors of the kitchen and Prana he breathed at night in his room on top story of a central Los Angeles skyscraper, levitated and experimented occasionally with smoking!

Klamonti's leading example is Mrs. Barbara Moore Pataleewa of London reported in June 17th, 1951, Sunday Chronicle. It said: "A woman of 50 who looks like she was only 30 claimed yesterday that she hates food, has beaten old age and expects to live at least 150 years. She has set out to do it by giving up eating. Twenty years ago she ate three normal meals a day. Slowly for 12 years she reduced her eating until she was keeping fit on one meal a day of grass, chickweed clover, dandelion, and an occasional glass of fruit juice. Five years ago she switched entirely to juices, raw tomatoes, oranges, grasses and herbs. Now she drinks nothing but a glass of water flavored with a few drops of lemon juice to kill the taste of chlorine. She says, "There is much more in sunlight and air than can be seen by the naked eye or by scientific instruments. The secret is to find the way to absorb that extra-that cosmic radiation-and turn it into food; that is what I have done. I am strong as any man, and need only four or five hours sleep for mental relaxation. Because I have no toxins in my system I am never ill. I had to advance gradually from vegetarianism to uncooked fruit and then to liquid food. Now I am struggling towards Cosmic Food. I have passed the eating stage and could not eat even if I desired, as my digestive apparatus has changed considerably and is now unable to handle any fiber at all. I now find the very smell of food disgusting." Your writer has used about the same method of transition in diet to give up eating, and I find the same true about the great discomfort experienced from the fiber in solid food. After reading some of Barbara's letters, I tried to correspond with her about similar naturist interests and Yoga in 1939, but her travels to Swiss Alps disrupted this. She does Yoga breathing and stands on her head daily.

More of the press reports given by Klamonti are: Feb. 6th, 1937 quote Mrs. Marthaq Nasch, age 44 of St. Paul, Minn. as asserting that for 7 years she had eaten nothing, and affirmed her willingness to submit to surveillance to prove her claim. May 31st, 1948 reports Yang Mel, age 20 investigated by Dr. T. Y. Gan of Chungking Municipal Hospital, to not have eaten for 9 years, shows no signs of starvation, leading a perfectly normal life except for having lost her desire for food and since her alimentary tract had become so dormant and rudimentary she could not take water anymore. A report of 1931 describes Mrs. Albert G. Walker, a noted singer of South Africa 101 days taking only water carrying on her singing while she reduced from 232 lbs. to 169 lbs., Jan. 25, 1938 states Biovanni Succi, traveling Europe giving exhibitions in 30 and 40 day fasts spent 8 years and 280 days without food in 10 years. Oct. 12th, 1948 reports a British girl of 12 years fasted 18 months taking nothing but water. John W. Armstrong of London fasted 100 days with water alone in 1932 regaining appearance of youth. Besides this information worthy of mention is report of Dr. Bernard Jensen: "A young woman seventeen years old by the name of Maria De Concieses from Mendes, Brazil, fasted 180 days or six months. She recovered from epilepsy with which she was afflicted. There was no great loss of weight, she remained very active and physicians found all organs perfect after the fast."

We are interested in information about others attempting non-eating, fasting, liquid and fruit diets as well as dedicate our service to sincere aspirants. Thus we announce the VITARIAN SOCIETY FOR CORRESPONDENCE AND INSTRUCTION IN FOODLESS LIVING. We do not wish to enlarge correspondence, but rather condense it to vitally practical aspirants, freeing time from answers to curiosity and elementary information which can obtained from other sources dedicated to same. Needless to say, one should have studied the lesson on Vitarianism preceding this, and be beyond the mere dreaming or theorizing stage of a diet free of seeds and animal proteins. As you have seen, complete abstinence takes years of persistence and patience in a gradual, but natural spontaneous transition.

Your writer made the journey from vegetarianism, thru the Vitarian fruit and vegetable diet, and semi-liquid fruit diet, to find it practical to give up eating on the tinctured water regimen (which we shall describe in a future lesson) after four months of encouraging results from the fall of 1952 to spring of 1953, so that there is someone to help you along if you are a sincere practising Vitarian. Spiritual Development is not a trick, magic, miracle or mystery but something attainable for persistent spiritual endeavor. Let us give to the world a Higher Spiritual Order of paradisical holymen of balanced spirituality, enjoying the enlightened contemplative life emancipated from the daily struggle to earn a living in the world, but not sustained by begging to be a burden on humanity because of their "holiness", rather than demonstrating magic and miracles that solve not the elementary problems of existence.

LESSON XIX

"THE AQUARIAN REGIMEN", NEW TINCTURED WATER APPROACH TO EFFORTLESS FASTING

The purpose of this lesson is to explain the "Aquarian Technique of Non-eating" or what may impersonally be called our Lord's message in the Spirit of Truth on the "Christian Effortless Path of Spontaneous Practical Spirituality." That this path can be relatively penanceless painless or the Golden Medium of Buddha (neither the worldly pleasures nor the other extreme of tortuous mortifications), or the natural effortless rhythm or order found throughout the universe, Lao-Tze said our life should conform to. Jesus Christ distinctly said His Yoga (Technique of Divine Yoking or Union) "is sweet and my burden light," Jesus, the Orient from on High, gave to the West the synthesis of all past knowledge and enlightenment of the culture thus far only developed in the East, as Luke 1 indicates, presenting a perfected teaching that would be the "Light of the world" which we might now refer to as the Christian Natural Yoga in the Serene Equilibrium of Love for Buddhic Wisdom. The burden (direct method to neutralize Karma) or the discipline in Christ is a hundredfold more effortless, painless or penanceless than required in effort for the illusory pleasures and things of the world, and the Yoga (Yoke) he asks us to learn of Him who is meek and humble of heart to endow Peace to our souls, is the Eternal Science of Immortality spoken of in the Bhagavad Gita, because Christian Natural Yoga is Life Everlasting.

Objection sometime arises to what some say is trying to save our mortal bodies, indicating its conflicts with Church teachings related to our bodies being sinful and evil and that we should instead mortify them. The teaching we give is not to save the mortal body for such is evil and sinful, death being the wages of sin. Like many other concepts of the new Truth Transcendent, the opposites are true. We must mortify the mortal body to save it, for it to put on immortality, for the spiritual resurrection of the flesh in God-birth in the Higher Kingdom. "The corruptible must put on the incorruptible and the mortal must put on the immortal." "know you not that your bodies are members of Christ", so "Glorify and bear God in your body." But to obtain this immortal and incorruptible Christ in body requires mortification, making die constantly the mortal and corruptible flesh. Immortality through mortification certainly not taught by anyone more than in our teaching of Penance, since besides abstinence from meat, excess food and stimulants on certain days like the Church, or periodic fasts on water, our new Aquarian or Water Regimen, is a perpetual washing or baptism of water for months or years till even water is abstained from. This constant killing of the old pleasure life of the mortal body for our Christ-Self gives constant resurrection of immortal flesh, cleanses one of morbidness in both body and mind, stagnation being death in material things. The mortal mind limits man by age limits, and other concepts while the Christ Mind is Immortal with its concepts in Life Everlasting. "Kill the mortal and cultivate the Immortal"! Matter has no permanent existence, being in constant change. But God, The Essence of All or the One Reality is everywhere in all things

Co-existent and this is the part to cultivate in our body, mind and soul when purging the mortal and corruptible.

Some people have tried to put on immortality merely by affirming it, and so far all these have died in spite of all their life believing they would not die! However, this is as fruitless as being "saved" by reading gospel tracts, because of believing one's self into Christ without rules He gave for Kingdom of God which is at hand. The Vitarian Philosophy established the foundation in the material body which is much more constant than the mortal mind which changes constantly with each moment's thought. In anybody the Spirit is willing, but the flesh is the weakness, so the real quest is overcoming the flesh and matter by applying the unchanging Cosmic Law or Christ's government, while the mind of man which has made its own rules ceases in its will and pursuits built on the sensual things. By Regenerating thru constant mortification we become like children in mental purity, free of morbid mortal feelings, not thinking, but feeling "We can live forever" because of the effervescent youth dynamically vibrating Life Everlasting and Immortal Christ in every cell of our incorruptible body, mind and soul. But we have to get at essentials, obtain the Vitarian Rejuvenescence of pre-puberty in corruptibility of the flesh, sealing the sex, eliminating the pathological growth of seed issue, thus destroying the desire, habit and need for material nourishment, sleep and other sensual pleasures that the concepts of good and evil are built on in our mortal mind. To those bound to the flesh, all this sounds like a tremendous thing to do, but from experience I tell you it is most effortless, spontaneous and the easiest path that comes natural if you seek close to Nature in God's Eternal Laws, not letting the world tempt you. At first, all man's troubles seemed a comedy, men enjoy them even at terrible cost, but how lamentable the sorrow and suffering coming from mental delusions. The mind and the senses only cast you astray, so contemplate Nature's revelation of this, as our Lord did, to seed eternal Truth and Substance in Christ-Law, Life and Light.

Even more people will question the mortification of the flesh, and the Holy Bible is being changed to mean that we need only to repent, and not do penance. It is argued that we are saved by Grace, not works, but why does one do the works of God except for Grace. For instance, I made a study of the Ecuadorean Saint Mariana's life which sounds more like mortification than living. Mariana was the proof of God's Grace, or what Easterners would call a good Karma earned by previous lives in virtue. Partial abstinence she started even while a baby, refusing nursing more than midday and evening and on Friday, Monday and Wednesday only once a day, refusing all attempts of extra feeding, but nevertheless she remained in good health. As a child she spent her time in prayer and penances, she shared Christ's passion on a cross made of five stones on the floor surrounded with nettles every Friday, she wore a penitential girdle of blackberry vines, and there were other "playmates" who became serious disciples in some of the agonies of the "via crusis". She even took up the hermit life on top of Mt. Pinchincha near Quito to pay homage to our Lady of Mercy, but God soon indicated this was not her path, along with another later plan to enter a Jesuit convent, but finally He showed His will to be for her to live the austere life of penance at home, not seeking elsewhere in the world. She meditated on death constantly, the inconsistency of life, the vanity of the world, and soon was sleeping 4 hours a night or less on a ladder, Friday night on a cross, besides walking with garbanzos in her shoes, wearing six blackberry vine girdles and fasted the whole week taking only one ounce of bread on Sundays. St. Mariana put up a battle unto death against flesh, outstanding among the virgin saints for having started it about 5 or 6 years of age and continued this taking the vow of perpetual chastity already past 8 years, and at 10, the vow of strictest poverty and obedience renouncing worldly pursuits. She was concerned with a need of greater things than even that rendered by Father Estaban at the time, who was the apostle of the Indians, there converting them by thousands and curing them of all manner of disease by laying of hands only. She defended this lashing and beating of her delicate body as though it were insensible, saying, "The greater the beating, the greater the delight in it"! But soon it came so that no matter how she beat and bled from wounds, which should have become as ulcers and give off odors ordinarily but now breathed out a sweet perfume, in the Holy Week they were healed instantly hiding all the butchery after the beatings.

She reduced her sleep to one hour daily, and, already in childhood having refused all animal foods including meats, fish,
eggs and milk in horror, she lived on a broth of cabbage leaves
and herbs, then one ounce of food till her stomach could take
none, and the last seven years of her life she ate no food,
using a little juice from an apple or other acid fruit to rinse her
mouth rarely but abstaining also from drinking water. It was
observed, however that her body would absorb water like
a blotter upon coming in contact with it in her surroundings.
Every opportunity the Saint had, she recommended fasting
to others, saying also that the greater the weakness felt, the
more endurance needed, the better the penance. In such little
space available here, little justice can be done for the virtues
of such saints as Mariana, the "Lily of Quito". She did not seek
pleasures even in ecstasy or phenomenal revelations, ever on
the firm path of self-denial and mortification (Luke 9:23;24).
Invoking sacrifice of her own life, she died (or suspended
animation of body) to stop the terrible earthquakes that were
shattering Ecuador in the seventeenth century. Her body remained flexible, like living, and giving off an aroma of flowers,
while many heard celestial music, which phenomena is also
recorded of oriental saints such as the great Yogi Milarepa of
Tibet. Six years after death the body was removed to another
burial spot but she was found beautiful in countenance as the
day she died, incorruptible to decay. This also happened with
her disciple Sebastian, who imitated her mortifications, 9 years
after death. Fearless, welcoming death constantly, death was
overcome till it was impossible for the body to die or decay.
This body incorruptibility is known of other Catholic mystics
and Oriental Yogis under the same procedure of mortification.
The lives of saints show how meager our efforts have been!
Most people rebel at the mention of it. Be patient, bear on with
me. Even science recently has discovered that in the wounds
of these saints, such as seen today by millions in Theresa
Neumann and others, is the very secret of the long sought
"seed of immortality"!

In the March 24, 1953, issue of "Look" magazine there
was an article "You May Live Forever", in which Wm. L. Laurence, the famed highest awards journalist connected with
Atomic discoveries, writes that Immortality, the constant

renewal of the physical body or the resurrection of the flesh is viewed as being very near at hand by science now. In re-search along this new frontier of life, Dr. Oscar Schotte dis-covered a universal law present wherever life manifests itself. Laurence writes: "the studies of Dr. Schotte have REVEALED THAT THERE EXISTS IN EVERY LIVING CREATURE, be it a tapeworm or a human being, THE SEED OF IMMORTALITY, a seed of the phoenix as it were, ENTIRELY DIFFERENT AND APART FROM THE EGG AND THE SPERM CELLS THAT GIVE RISE TO OFFSPRING in the normal perpetuation of the species. This newly discovered seed of perpetual life, verily the fountain of youth sought thru the ages, has been identi-fied by Dr. Schotte as the regenerative scar tissue that keeps the body in constant repair thru-out life and without which life would be much shorter than it actually is. It is these very phoenix cells, molded by the sculptor of life, that rebuild every cell and organ in our body, with exception of our brain and central nervous system, about every seven years. When man has at last succeeded in definitely isolating the sculptor and in determining the sort of tools and working conditions it requires, -goals scientists universally agree will definitely be reached in the not-too-distant future,-man will have learned the secret of immortality." Now these modern scientists, without giving any credit to the mystic, are going to "isolate the sculptor of life", and in the essential step which "is a very simple thing" by keeping some cells of scar tissue cells by quick freezing or tissue culture by proper nutrient, they will have a mythical "Phoenix Nest" for renewing human bodies. They think they can just take the omnipotent Creator of life, putting Him in a laboratory test tube, and keep thus "indefinitely in a state of perfect preservation, the spark of life in a state of suspended animation, yet ever ready to spring into life"! We do hope and pray that they really isolate the Intelligent Spirit governing all life from matter in their perception of Truth, and do not create a laboratory hell for thousands of innocent animals, as they have fumbling with the manifestation of disease without seeking its Cause. However, their studies do have facts valuable in prov-ing Vitarianism to others.

First we have emphasized in capitals above, the seed of immortality or regeneration and healing is distinct from the seed of mortality or generation and what sexologist Dr. Rutgers termed an "embryonic tumor" intermediary between growth and pathological tumors removed by surgeons. This fact disproves the claims of past conclusions of both the scientists and the mystics, for the Vitarian Insight, as to the generative fluids. The scientist has held that a moderate use of the sex was essential to body health condoning sexual passion as a means of enriching life, and mystics, especially Yoga teachers, though saying one should not waste the fluids only erroneously claimed this was done to conserve the substance and energy that would be re-absorbed, or transmuted only to be frustrated by the scientist who proved that semen could not be re-absorbed for such claims. Our teaching began with the pointing out of the need to eliminate menstruation, pollutions and sexual generative fluid production, to conform to the universal law of regeneration observed in plants which keep on perpetuating themselves if one prevents them from going to seed, besides the theory in Steinach operation which we claimed failure as much as celibate's theorized re-absorption to prevent losses that could only result in protein decomposition of albuminuria and uric acid toxic-poisoning in the blood. We don't assimilate food to produce body cells, much less semen, though these both can be re-absorbed in the form of stimulating irritants to habitually give degenerate feelings of well-being. Dr. Carrel showed that the cell was immortal, perpetuated itself by renewal and not by nourishment, as long as correct washing solution was renewed. Prof. Huxley showed how injurious feeding was to living things, by fasting earthworms to make them live 19 generations (or more if there be patience given) beyond the ordinary life span, also showing that the key to producing more seed of immortality and diminishing the seed of mortality in generative fluids, was in fasting baptisms of body cells, as much as the healing propensity created by the infliction of wounds calling forth the dormant Creative Faculty lost or atrophied by non-use after the body growth ceases and sheltered civilized life stagnates it. Athletes know use builds muscles, and not the eating of animal muscles. The hard knocks of football and the constant beating of the boxer make him hard thru and thru. The cracking of the barefoot soles, the prostrations of postures of prayer, tedious labor, hard bed besides the extreme silence make the ascetic impervious to the accelerated aging common to those living in the comforts of the world. Wear and tear of the body were erroneously assumed to destroy the body, since they only keep our creative healing powers from atrophying from stagnation, and often we hear the testimonial from people over a century in age claiming their longevity to keeping active always. Age and death can thus directly be attributed to partaking in pleasures rather than work and constructive efforts which man dislikes and thus pins his troubles to, and first in these habitual pleasures is eating substances that become irritants and stimulants that waste the body tissue, first manifesting in puberty producing the tumorous growth of generative cells, the seed of mortality.

These new studies in the science of "Phoenixology" (as Laurence terms it) also give us the recognized authoritative secular backing of science on the revelation of the "Mystery of Life" symbolized in the mystic crucifix. Jesus demonstrated how the path of non-violence and love to all in the Divine will overcome all material obstacles in this world if we will pay our debts in penance till it is physically impossible to suffer more. Certainly a great amount of scar tissue must have been produced as He was beaten, maimed, whipped, crowned with thorns and finally nailed on the cross, so as to be a complete bruise all over, requiring a complete seed of immortality regeneration of every bit of the body which happened in three days to give the completely reborn body, perfected even to the capability of Ascension. The deathless state, He showed, came by a resurrection thru Love, not hating his enemies and attackers, forgiving their actions to the last moment because they knew not what they were doing and not succumbing to poisoning his pure blood with glandular toxins that otherwise kill a man thru anger, fear and hate. Paying the penalties for sin, mortals become Immortals right here on earth. He did not tell us we had to do the same thing He did, but demonstrated that no matter how extreme the burden in sin, and He chose to bear ours with us, if we conform to God's Will to the very last degree. Salvation is secure above all things. Such a Path of the Cross carried on over a period of years in a Discipline He laid down to His disciples, would be very light and sweet to carry for our Lord.

"Now if Vitarianism is so VITAL, why didn't Jesus teach it so specifically and definitely as you do?" is a question that is put to your writer. Jesus did the most revolutionary thing in his era as it was, and to cast the pearls of Wisdom to those who would hate and reject them and Him all the more, was then untimely. The Scriptural students, preachers and priests of his time said to Him, "You don't know enough to observe God's commandment on how to keep our Sabbath, you defend an adulteress rather than obey the commandments of Moses that she be stoned, you reject your father and mother in public rather than honor them, you violate the commandments of our faith in worship and now you call yourself the Son of God! Crucify this blasphemer!" However, this was the very mission of Christ at that time, and as Paul wrote to the Hebrews VIII:7-13, He gave us a new Covenant in which He reflected these precepts and traditions of the men of old, and as prophesied He gave God's laws into their minds and into the hearts of men, and the Spirit of Truth will teach us all things. OF THE PATH, Paul goes on to say, "A new and living way which he hath dedicated for us, thru the veil, that is to say, his flesh...Let us draw near with a true heart in fullness of faith, having our hearts sprinkled from an evil conscience, and OUR BODIES WASHED WITH PURE WATER." Baptism means not only by immersion but includes internal washing.

However, the time was not ripe during the first two thousand years of the Christian era for the Spirit and Water Baptism Penance of the New Aquarian Age, and rejecting the lighter yoke, the Saints have taken the more violent Baptism of Blood penances of Martyrdom like Jesus characterized for the Piscean Age.

Now the word "Jesus" has the meaning especially mystically traced Iesous, or icthus, pisces, fish related to feet or the foundation of all. Jesus (fish) went to the submerged depths of the sea of men (multitudes), bringing up the first disciples in fishermen, whose feet he washed in humble Oneness and fed the multitudes "fish". It is the understanding created by the last phrase of the sentence that has perpetuated the eating of flesh foods by ordinary Christians, much to their sensual liking, and thus kept up the need for bloodshed and wars, in spite of the teaching of Peace. Some Protestant Bibles have even added that Jesus ate the pascal lamb, besides fish, since they wanted to clarify to people that penances such as abstinence from meat like the Saints, besides certain periods for the Church were not in order. The Catholic Rheims version states that after the resurrection "Jesus cometh and taketh bread, and giveth them and fish in like manner" not saying He ate the food though He did distribute it for them, but all this came in a miraculous manner though the disciples had no fish to begin with till he made the abundance available from spiritual resources which needs no killing for that is its law. Now in feeding the 5,000 men, Rheims states, "He took the five loaves and the two fishes and looking up to heaven, he blessed and brake, and gave the loaves to his disciples and the disciples to the multitudes, and they did all eat and were filled." We note thus he gave them only loaves. The Essenes to whom He belonged, according to many authorities, were a vegetarian sect "fanatic" about living the first law of God that man's food was herb and fruit, in their ritual used a sacrificial offering of loaves shaped like fish, rather than the slaughtered carcasses of animals and fish like Jews, so thus he took ordinary loaves and fish-shaped with same Aramaic name of fish, and created astral dream matter from these, gave the duplication to all, which released their minds from the sensual desire of eating by the symbolic fishes precipitated from the thin air. And what would it matter if he fed them ordinary tasting fish of no material substance for a spiritual miracle, since the law is not broken thus as to killing natural creatures. We should not believe in the visions, but in the gospel and laws He taught, since man's visions can hypnotically relate him to own desires always. "Destroy not the works of God for flesh". Throughout the Scriptures can be found instances supporting the Vegetarian Essene teaching, and especially is this emphasized in Vatican Aramaic scrolls, file record No, 156-P, written by John Beloved in which Christ commands "Kill neither men, nor beasts, nor yet the food that goes in your mouth" prescribing live food only. From the majority of the first Christians being vegetarians, it is evident this was the Essene teaching among the disciples, though the secular part of the Church suppressed this teaching. Jesus had to get to the hearts of men with teachings of vast scope without creating rejection by food habits, but when asked (Mark II) why He did not fast though he taught this, He indicated when He is taken away "then they shall fast in those days" besides giving the parable of putting new wine in new bottles only to explain that fasting was for the new order to come later, though not fitting for His time, disciples or Him. Today the sacrifice of animals has been given up and the vegetarian diet is recognized by all men as beneficial at least, and the new Aquarian abstinence from food and "Aqua" (water) or Aquarian Rule of Discipline is given.

The Piscean Age was that of blood-bearing in which literally martyrs were redeemed in the blood of Jesus Christ, with the Baptism of blood and death for Salvation, but the Aquarian Age is that of water-bearing, continuing the Teachings of John the Baptist in the Water Baptism, and Jesus Christ in Spirit of Truth Baptism for which both were killed, to give man the deathless regeneration and translation besides the liberated Foodless Living. Our "Eternal Youth Life" message No. 1 from Ecuador on Sept. 13, 1946, came out with the revelation that our mission was effectuating the New Age, Order and Race of the Heavenly Kingdom redeeming mankind from the two millenniums of the bloody purification by martyrs, crusades, Stigmata wounds, and such to an "Eternal Youth Life" of esthetic beauty in Christ consciousness. Your writer returned to the U.S. " to the world again in the Spirit of John the Baptist, teaching men to make ready their living temples for the Coming of the Lord, by fasting and prayer" for a "Renaissance of the Pristine Perfection." Christ's Basic Requirement, "Unless a man be born again of water and the Holy Spirit, he cannot enter the Kingdom of God," necessarily means a life from water and Spiritual Union till the body is completely re-created eliminating all thirst for worldly existence and the translation, ascension or complete absorption into the Father, Supreme Omniscient Spirit.

By this time you are probably ready to listen to personal experiences rather than being "bored" with so much philosophy! The record is humiliating, out of 18 years experience as a vegetarian, about 7 years were on an exclusive fruit diet, and after returning to California the completion of this lesson is with only 7 month living without eating on the Aquarian Regimen.

Yet I already knew about living without eating besides acquiring an ideal in it, 15 years ago, and within a few months then I had broken all ties and was in ideal conditions for the transition in California, living on a juicy fruit diet, in a year practically next to goal on the semiliquid diet of oranges, but chasing visions and ideals that took me away from the goal, I fumbled away time in experiments of altitudes, diets, penances, and other aspects far off in the Andies. This deviation may be justified in the attainment of the last 10 years of God-Consciousness, but finally all the philosophizing on life without eating has become embarrassing enough to "make one move from one chair to another to avoid the draft!" Had the 33 years of this incarnation been conveyed by understanding from a comprehensive study of the subject as given in Vitarianism here within, the time could have been reduced to no more than 3 years for a normal young person from any kind of diet for the transition. Such is the struggle and bewilderment of the rational sense-bound mind in spiritual pursuits! But see how merciful the Lord has been in spite of all the fumbling, how patiently He bears our weak will, and how effortless the Way.

Spiritual Baptism is into the body by drinking, meaning the water baptism is likewise besides a pre-requisite as evidenced throughout our Scriptures (I-Cor.12:13, Acts 2:38, Jn. 3:5). The new discovery that will revolutionize future efforts to live without eating is in a more or less spontaneous natural transition from the fruit diet to what I call THE TINCTURED WATER REGIMEN AVERAGING 1% NUTRITION DERIVED FROM ACID FRUIT JUICE DILUTED IN 99% WATER. Ultimately this technique prepares the digestive tract as it gradually and naturally is atrophied for the complete abstinence from both food and drink which is a transition much more abrupt than in diet changes, removing the greater part of the stomach and abdomen so that the muscles, organs and various parts have to be re-created, and after a new fashion. Primarily the minutely flavored water enables one to consume much greater quantities of water, necessary for the constant internal baptism of the body, than can be taken if it is ordinary, tasteless, cold water as usually practiced in fasting. Fasting sanatorium physicians will argue about this trifle, saying that if any food, no matter how minute the quantity of juice of acid fruit containing so little substance that may be claimed of any food value, does not activate the digestive functions, hunger, showing that at a certain degree of dilution digestibility is lost no matter how much be consumed. Moreover, the fact that one can go on indefinitely fasting on tinctured water, still proves that all the theories of food values, need of adequate protein, carbohydrates, minerals, etc.., are false and that the body is not built out of food. As revolutionary as Christ's message to the physicians, the Vitarian Philosophy declares that equally deceptive as the many pharmaceutical medicines sold to the public to deaden the pains of disease advancing in the body, are the many new miracle foods, nutritional supplements and concentrates now advertised in Health magazines which are nothing but sales catalogs composed of testimonials on food discoveries. Both Medical and Naturopathic doctors base the nutritional needs of man on Medical Research in laboratories experimenting with rats, monkeys and sometime the degenerate civilized creature called man. However, all foods are stimulants, habit forming, and used to balance the abdominal poisoning already going in the body. Mainly, as Jesus told men centuries ago, food purges the flesh rather than defiles it, since each time man eats he pushes out the decomposing ferment rotting in the intestines so that it will not poison man . Now you can take pills, alkaline foods and what not to neutralize somewhat the poison brewing in there, or you may go on the famous cure of saints, nature doctors, and known instinctively by animals, by which I refer to fasting.

But in ordinary fasting you take only water and the filthy mess in the intestines, some of it with an age of many years found cemented in pockets of the intestines, remains there being absorbed into the blood in the form of toxins, mucous, etc., that given one headaches, heavily coated tongue, bad circulation sensible to temperatures, "weakness" or rather paralysis of muscles form a toxic blood, etc. So the ordinary procedure of fasting calls for the use of an enema which in practice only gets to lower part of the descending colon doing practically nothing to really clean the entire 5 feet of the colon which in 7-8ths of the human  family is filled with hardened encrusted matter besides maggots and pus in cases. Even with a clean colon, using a 1.5 foot flexible rubber catheter on the enema tube, one has to get the transverse colon lower than rectum, helping water around to the ascending colon, if capable with Yogic intestinal contractions, and with 3 to more injections of water repeated. Rather than this work-out with the country type of high enema, most people will rather pay the high prices asked for a "Colonic" that force the water in. But suppose you clean the last 5 feet of the intestines of the colon, there still remains the remainder of the intestinal canal which is over 30 feet long, besides the digestive tract up thru the stomach to the mouth that while you were eating was being thoroughly cleansed by the passage of food. If you drink a little water it does not wash this out since plain water is mucous-repellent and goes out thru to the kidneys leaving the insides of the faster filthy. Even after years of a fruit diet there are some residues that collect all along digestive tract and intestines that have to be cleansed or bathed daily in the macrocosmic human body, just like in the microcosmic cell which the famed Nobel awards surgeon, Dr. Carrell, said was immortal needing only renewal of the fluid it is bathed with. Eventually, we can learn to adjust to needing no water, condensing it from the air, but meantime the transition needs to be smooth without insurmountable amounts of obstacles piled up to overcome. One thing at a time; we shall attend to all without dismay of our task nor complications to confuse us.

Consequently, our regimen uses an internal wash water tinctured with juice from acid fruits which act as a solvent for mucous on the tongue, and all along the digestive and intestinal tract. In Florida we used to wash our clothes with tart seedling oranges, lemons, etc., and grapefruit was especially good for the hair and general bathing...Nature's own detergent growing on a tree! Internally, on the tinctured water I found lemon juice too harsh, and even on tender skin burning can be felt if it is used as an antiseptic. Beginning the regimen, the first month I used a 2% ratio of nutrition to 98% water taking the water three times a day, just like I had taken 3 meals a day on the exclusive fruit diet for 7 months preparatory to this. This habitual rhythm is always a good rule to follow in changes, and too many students think that they must gather together all their obstacles and reforms, and with one big smash with all their will power they will conquer all, a Master of all in one trial! This

kind of ambition is too easily defeated. So in the regimen I
used tomato juice added to a four fifths part of boiling water
to homogenize the mixture, followed by light spearmint tea
flavored with pure sorghum syrup for the cold mornings and
evenings of December and January, and Navel orange juice
diluted in water at midday. The tea following the tomato juice is
optional, remnant of the "dessert" habit, though the spearmint,
of a spearmint-Chamomile herb combination which is abundantly wild here and the writer's favorite, destroys body acids
in the wash, and the Sorghum syrup should be 100% pure,
light and not dark like molasses, which is used on machine
belts, and not fragrant. This is the best sweetener we have
found outside sugar in fruit, found in groceries, and not filled
with mineral matter, that Vitarianly speaking, pollutes the black
strap molasses health potions, and since we seek not digestibility but least irritating flavor for water, we are not concerned
over dextrose-phobia, though honey we would shun more for
enslaving bees besides the formic acid that burns throat in
those not used to it. But the second month we decided to eliminate all vegetable sugar flavor and reduce the proportions of
the tincture 1% nutrition to 99% water. Even the tomato juice
from cans was eliminated, using a raisin tea made by adding
a couple of large spoonfuls of chopped seedless raisins to
a quart of boiling water supplementing spearmint, if desired,
which gives a tart rather than sweet tea as imagined perhaps
for the sugar dilution being beyond digestibility, and with it I
used the Navel orange juice flavored water. However, by this
time the Navel orange of February was tree ripe, and contained too much sugar with little acid to aid intestinal cleansing, and with readily assimilable sugar some was assimilated
bringing back hunger, the flow of digestive juices, so I could
not get mind off drinking little more water than necessary and
after three weeks experiments trying to adjust to apparently
more ideal source I returned to the old stand-by of tomato juice
diluted now one part juice to 10 parts water, or 99.5% water
with one half of 1% nutrition. All this time I was using at least
one gallon of water daily.

Then the beginning of Lent, thinking it auspicious, I
tried to discontinue even the taking of water, nothing entering
the mouth, but after 7 days the body was weak, the muscles

dehydrated and paralyzed just like when I fasted 40 days on water only or when I had beri-beri in the jungle unable to continue caring for myself. I tried various things, such as breathing aromatic vapor in room all day which increased urine one pint per day, showing possibilities of vapor condensation in humid countries and tropics, nor are non-eaters known to exist in deserts in my observations. The bowel movements on correctly tinctured water continue at least once a day, constantly removing all wastes from mouth to colon, but on the dry fast with no movement, the stagnant residues on the mucous membranes in a week gave nausea from coated tongue, the acid in stomach may have caused sensibility felt there, the toxins in the intestines sent toxins to the brain causing headaches of a lesser degree besides the muscular paralysis in spite of my years of pure diet, and it persisted in spite of attempting high enemas. After my experiments with 40 day and 24 day fasts and 12,000 feet elevation under all ideal conditions, this problem of washing the intestines prevented me from achieving the goal in non-eating, since this is a prime factor. It is not natural to force water up backwards thru the alimentary canal nor does that wash out encrusted residues, nor can water from the mouth be taken in sufficient quantity to wash inside any amount without fruit acids which are naturally called for to dissolve the mucous and other waste and carry it to be eliminated from the body. Water drinking in the fast only carries sticky mucous and waste of digestive tract dumping it 30 feet short of elimination in the small intestines where drinking water is absorbed, and no colonic wash ever invented can get it, to prevent it from being absorbed as more poisoning for the blood from an increasingly potent ferment! Herewithin lies the physiological factor contributing to the wonderful results from the new system of the Aquarian revelation.

So from there on I continued in patient persistence to an indefinite time, within the next three years probably, as has always been the case with the other foodless livers of our research, that the body naturally finds it has no use for the constant internal bathing and water drinking can be given up also along with the elimination of eating. Leaving off from the fruit diet was unabrupt, spontaneous under spiritual influences of Divine Oneness with our Lord, just as the fruit diet is just naturally more appetizing and less bother and effect than using fruit and vegetable salads in the Vitarian diet, which is a reformed Vegan comprehension, eventually advanced to after beginning vegetarianism. Patience and persistence must be used in each transition of greater abstinence of food habits, till the regimen becomes a "second nature", preventing losing all ground gained so far, and the organism progresses to the necessary purification. After many months of experience I found it best to stick to a 1% nutritionally valued tincture of acid fruit juice diluted in 99% water. This can be obtained by homogenizing (boiling into) one part tomato juice, five or six parts water and to avoid monotony of same thing constantly, this can be flavored in a new "broth" each time by just a pinch of herbs such as parsley, basil, celery, etc., that must be strained out afterward, just like the raisins from the tea water, so that no fiber or vegetable paste of any kind get into the system. Some students concoct a theory that they will use an herb broth transition, which will fill the intestines with an encrusted paste and give worse results than a good live food regimen with roughage to sweep out insides. After living many years on nettle broth, secluded, nearly naked and practicing ascetic meditation, like all great teachers that come back later to give the world a great teaching, Milarepa, the Yogi-Saint of Tibet, broke his nettle broth pot on a rock, out of which rolled a perfect green image formed from the hardened encrustations of nettle broth froth, which he took as an auspicious symbol to return to the world to teach disciples, since the old earthy form had given out completely for the inner form accumulated from a well ordered life of discipline! Nettles are of the tastiest cooked vegetables to add as a dressing for a salad in an elementary Vitarian diet but not in Non-eating if you don't want a green image accumulating inside, and on it weakness comes surprisingly to the inexperienced thinking it's little more nourishment that would help. In March the Spring orange was still acid, but worked fine for the tincture for not having sugar content of tree-ripe Navels, and when they are too sweet the grapefruit comes in. What matters is that one take in enough water to wash out the system completely, with enough acid to carry a small amount of liquid residue to the bowels for a movement each day, and that the tincture be non-assimilable for being too diluted to activate digestive functions with a liquid part in solvent fruit acids that cleanse but do not become absorbed in the intestines like most of the water. Even on ordinary diets people wither away if they don't get enthusiastic about them, since shunning their food they don't get the needed water and dry up (body and food both mostly water) and refusal to eat enough of the new reformed diet does not push out intestinal wastes so autointoxication sets in and new diet makes them sick, but eating enough, even on a fruit diet keeps one fat in flesh. Your writer is not fat on this, nor plump like other Non-eaters of years duration, but I am able to continue all my work, cultivating a garden to give to friends (like Theresa Neumann cultivates flowers for the altar), cut firewood for heating in winter, mimeograph all the output of the one-man Publications, edit the magazine, attend correspondence, etc., all of which would take several office employees, besides spiritual contemplative insight and prayer work at night. The net result was greater efficiency and sublimer spiritual accomplishments. All non-eaters were very active or did rigorous breathing for this.

Jesus took His disciples to the top of a Mount for prayer and His sermon, which is a Natural Deep Breathing cleansing, just like Yogic Pranayama precedes Meditation, however artificially assimilated into their technique. Natural outdoor activity is a great strength-builder, and Mountain climbing aids ecstatic God-Contemplation. Ecstatic Breath developed in god-Raptures is the third Breatharian technique. Jesus did not profane virginal relationships in spontaneous Love among individuals, commanding memorial of His annointings by Mary Magdalene by it being preached as part of the gospel. His Way of Life He supported by Nature Contemplation, saying, "Consider the lilies of the field," etc., explaining how we should abandon worldly pursuits for riches, food, clothing, homes, jobs enslaving us to material seekings and being bound to family relationships and the world. His Integral Naturism as the direct, spontaneous and highest way to live in God-Dedication was the Supreme Light that excelled His teaching above the Enlightenment of past teachers. Man does not like to find this in the bible, preferring rituals, tradition, ceremonies in churches and schemes of theoretic knowledge to avoid living (the) truth. Life itself, in every action, becomes one's religion in practice with Christ Nature the school, and the place that we worship is the wide open spaces!

## LESSON XX LEMURIAN GENESIS, HELIOIVORA THAT DID NOT EAT, TINCTURE WATER CHART

To get a truer idea of the God-perfected man of the new race of the Resurrection or the renewed Celestial Kingdom of the new earth, we find it necessary to reconstruct the story of God-created man of the original golden race of the Golden Age. This takes us back to the old Mother continent "Mu" or Lemuria where a superior civilization dwell of which now in the depths of the Pacific Ocean are found great cities with great highways extending hundreds of miles and many immense stone structures that completely baffle our science, now sunken with parts above here and there remaining on some Pacific isles. This was the home of the original hermaphroditic man told of in Genesis I in the "generation of heaven and earth," who was created in the image of God and that this race of man was bisexual is proven in the words, "Male and female He created them." And God blessed them enabling them to "increase and multiply" without sin, but as they came in God's image they materialized a number of bodies from rarefied substance thru the Light of God, like the Yogis who even today can multiply bodies thru control of Life-force "Prana". Certainly to bring man to this planet and transport beings to other planets, God did not need man-made space-ships as our modern man might theorize. In fact, after our planet was broken away from the sun and thru aeons of time became inhabited by what we may classify higher beings, it was without the ordinary atmosphere we breathe, requiring a "helioivora" power of sustenance as well as the Helios or sun-substance.

Much of this lesson will shock the reader in its completely unheard of assertions made from direct contact with the Spirit of Truth Transcendent, just as was attempted by the ancient sages, prophets and Christ, and let us be patient to feelings of credulity or incredulity for sometimes contradicting secular information, besides seemingly correcting what people think was the teaching of prophets like Moses and even clarifying the Christ-Doctrine given by the Apostles. Bear with me, it

is not dead prophets that can produce living Truth form revelation. Too often "the letter killeth". Cautiously shall I say, the
original Son God created on earth was not "Breatharian" nor
was He "Fruitarian" or "Vitarian", but in the male and female
completeness the godly humans were completely sustained
only by the sun's rays or "Helioarian".

Note the use of the suffix "arian" used for occupation,
culture or character and origin of root meanings connect this
with "Aryan" as nobility, culture and character. The term "Aryan", describing the Indo-European or Indo-Germanic languages, refers to the race of Caucasian people coming west and
going south to a country they called "Arya" (India) from the
"Cradle of Humanity" attributed to Central Asia, which was
originally populated from Lemurian migration. The first particular branch in Aryan nobleness ever created was the "cult",
which means worship, of their "culture" of cultivated sunliving
or "Helio-Aryan-ism", that later was referred to in Hebrew
Scriptures and else-where as "Sun-Worshipping" and characterized all Aryans in common origin. Inhabiting high plateaus,
the first Helio-Aryans did have the ability to live from the sun's
rays, but desires in the use of God-Given creative powers
they endowed themselves with a paradise of pleasures first
of beauty in green vegetation to clothe the bleak earth that
blossomed into aromatic flowers and delicious fruits, and then
eventually of utility after the development of lungs and stomach in man. Though the Helioarians absorbed the solar energy
direct thru their translucent skin just as we still get some of our
life energy such as Vitamin D, and like the plants absorb their
power of life in photo-synthesis, organs we call the lungs were
developed to absorb more of the dense but organically aromatic air that came about when the plant life started to transform
the ozone of our rarefied atmosphere into oxygen to give off
the solar atomic energy of life to operate the plant's chlorophyll
factory. (03-02 = energy release). Thus now it is with greater
difficulty that man lives from the denser air surrounding his organic paradise, requiring a special ecstatic breath to recharge
body vitality if he abstains from food completely, whereas the
first man found ozonated air plentiful just as still found in the
super-altitude air where man naturally loses his desire and
need to eat.

The later statement may I support with my study of attempts to climb Mt. Chimborazo in Ecuador, which showed that the climbers lost all desire and ability to sleep or eat in the snowy super-altitudes, so that in all practical honesty, I have had intentions to adapt to living in the snow like the polar explorer, where the air would naturally sustain the body. This I explained to the U.S. Consul in Quito when I was trying to determine God's Will as to the next move from Lake Quilo-toa when the 7 month 7 day initiatory period was concluded, considering that; 1. I could come back to U.S. in obligation to humanity to give out the new teachings facing the threat of an Atom War as a Pacifist, 2. I could teach disciples in Quito who showered offers of convenience and publication facility on me, or 3. I could realize my personal desire in seeking spiritual extreme by going to live in the snows of Mt. Chimborazo, the earth's supreme altitude. His argument that I could do much for mankind, judging from the British and other foreign articles printed on my hermit life, I answered that more could be done thru prayer or human telepathically than with teaching which builds resistance from imperfect words and that since God, Christ or Life was Omnipresent, it would sustain one even on Chimborazo's top as elsewhere. In the end he bid me bon voyage saying if I wasn't careful I'll be a very famous man which only robbed my hopes in ideal in principles that are unpopular with men.

Thus the "Helio-Aryans" lost their true nobility or culture to become merely a cult, or gave up the sun-practice culture for a mere sun-worshipping religion and migrating to denser air of low valleys and farther away from the equator, and took to wearing clothes rather than absorbing sunlight thru their translucent skin as do plants, and naturists notice to contain factors that can eliminate half our food. But the customs of Sun-day worship, Sun-rise religious services, sun-set prayer, solstice or sun festivals, etc., continued with the Aryan race adoring the sun of the sun, Light of lights, Life of all life at the altar of the visible sun in thankfulness for God's Light, Love and Life given thru this source contemplated in the sun.

The "Breath-Aryans" took their culture to India establishing the Yoga Science of Breath and spiritual Culture, and to this day there are some practical enough in this to live or sustain themselves from the technique of Life they teach in the lower valleys of the Himalayas. Breatharians take their food from the nitrogen and other gases, besides the bacteria and microbes that abound in the dense jungle air from decomposing vegetation, besides the oxygen from the process of photosynthesis in plants. Notice how many of the cases of non-eaters we mentioned in our previous lessons live at low altitudes in India, Bavaria, etc. But I think some of the Breatharians of the Jain Life conserving philosophy not only feel that they should avoid walking on God-created grass, not to speak of worms, bugs, etc. (that St. Francis and Buddha removed from any path) and thus sought not to destroy Life in the air they breathe. Doing deep breathing absorbing great quantities of air, just as much microscopic plant life besides the microscopic organism similar to taking milk or mushrooms. Thus Breatharians seek high altitudes for more solar energy, to destroy the least amount of organic Life in the air and thus enjoy the Heliorian Bliss of Perfection in the Infinite Interchange of Innermost Intimacy with the Initial Intelligence of Existence. All that is given to Life is returned more abundantly, our Being in God a channel of Blessing.

Genesis contains truth inspiration, though it may have gotten to us at times out of chronology perhaps due to the conditioned reason when it was written from observing each new day bring visibility of plants on earth without seeing the sun. But how could the trees and herbs of the 3rd day of creation exist since all life depends on solar radiations that were not created till the 4th day. Just as each new translation of the Bible censors it with new facts or fancies of men of each generation, we have to depend in the end on our own God-contact in spite of its inspirational authority. Personally, I feel the helioarian man is first rather than after the fruit and herbs on earth, which living as a true son of God he got thru mental creation, however, from a proud feeling of free-will separate from the Creator in his curiosity and power, making him soon dependent on a Fruitarian and Vitarian existence. That animals devolved from man in structure rather than vice versa which in turn only accounts for man's evolution in soul, can be seen before our eyes. Man cannot evolve apes into men by breeding,

though human babies taken to be mothered by apes degenerate into apes in characteristics completely, just as men degenerates into brutes becoming "animalistic" thru disobedience
to God's Law of life, but are resurrected into sainthood and
greater power in wisdom above all else thru God's Government is his life. Renouncing God for free-will he lost his power
of Omniscience and became a slave, beast of burden and so
on lower perpetuating the material rather sustenance in nature
than seeking Truth in Spirit that would make beings free as is
the eventual Goal of all creation.

We are challenged in our statements that man originally did not need fruit, herb for meat or food (Gen. 1:29), since
we would say that eating is only a habit for pleasure which
God gave to Adam and the rest of Lemurians as a blessing
and not as a commandment to eat as was the case with immaculate conception for birth, by those who say: "It is natural
for man to eat because he has teeth." Our answer is that we
question this reasoning saying it is neither originally natural for
man to eat nor to have teeth. Man is not born with teeth! Man
has to develop teeth after birth and go thru a teething process,
and readily loses them in a diet change besides from later
bad nourishment, showing them not intended as a permanent
perfect part but acting in makeshift to accommodate his habits.

When a baby is born to a mother who lives on an
unnatural diet, it is attached to the nourishment it got from her
blood, and thus it has to be suckled with an adapted secretion
of her blood from her breast. After cannibalism, sucking from
the blood of its own kind, it goes to carnivorous sucking from
animal mammary secretions and because nature is trying to
adapt to the dietary habits of the mother and of a cow, teeth
develop in the child, but again they prove inadequate when the
change is made to conventional dietary habits, so the "milk"
teeth come out for new ones. Later they are always a weak
link in man's makeup, already in early teens school children
show a 90% development of caries and even the Indians living
on natural whole grains such as the early Zunis had tooth decay 75% for the need of a gizzard in man.

Some may object saying babies look ugly and to be

"toothless" is fitting only for the aged. However, this standard is based on familiarity, and we might appreciate the baby smile if all lived without eating like the original hermaphroditic humans who lived as "sons of God" in a baby's innocence compared to the modern man equipped with natural or artificial "grave-diggers." Now the carcass-fed over-stuffed "human" gleams happily at all around him showing the canine or dog teeth developed on his vicarious feeding from animal proteins obtained by cruel enslavement of beasts, while fondly esteeming the morbid utterances of "Drop dead", "Were we drunk", "They'll tar and feather him", "That little piggy became pork sausage", etc.!

How much more esthetic is the serene compassionate smile of Buddha and of Mona Lisa! True beauty needs only the loving smile of kindness, serene and sympathetic, while the grin showing the threatening human fangs he develops after his feeding from animal substance and sensual stimulant not only portrays man's irresponsible feelings in killing and war besides carnal pleasures, but also resembles the grave welcome from Death's skull as he grins indulgently at man's record of sins marked in his suicidal weapons hiding in his own mouth!

Also, originally the Helio-Aryan bodies were of more rarefied material than ours, but this man, intuitionally-enlightened image of God that he was, thru tempting power and curiosity desired continually to know matter to a greater extent which contact resulted in a gradual absorption of it so as to increase the body's density and give colors to the races according to the excess of the more lifeless inorganic substance that also made it more opaque or lightless. Black is the absence of color, brilliant white light containing all the colors, just as the white race is the fullness of complete racial experience having blended or melted in the other race colors.

Food substance is known to color the skin and hair as much as any other factor. Fruitarians eating papayas for years get an orange tinge in their skin while Tibet's Yogi-saint Milarepa living years in seclusion on no more than nettle broth as food, became green-tinged in skin and hair. So originally the way of life gave the divisions in race pigmentation. The African cannibal took on the black skin of death from the corpses they ate and even psychically inflicted as heredity in their offspring. The brown savage living on the carcass of animals took on their color and characteristics while less guilt is reflected in the Eskimo's skin color where plant food is scarce, as well as the Jews, Mohammedans who abstain from hog meat. Also, the excessively starchy and cooked diet giving much carbon and calcareous mineral materials drawn into hair and skin pigmentation by a hot tropical sun, colors the Latin American and Oriental Indian since travelers observe the succeeding generations of the same race in the high Himalayas or Andies become white like Europeans, which evaluates the more ozonated air of altitudes and coniferous forests. The yellow race living in crowded lands as Japan and China, do not have other nitrogen or humus to put into the soil to grow crops than the excrement of man and beast giving an excessive uric acid content from centuries of accumulation, which also gives their yellow complexion. Certainly the hereditary factor has much to do with a child who nourished from mother's blood and reflects the expressions of the parents in a psychic influence also, but after the fourth generation one race disappears in among others if the physical causes cease.

The Lemurians planted the ozone generating Sequoia trees in the California, Sierra Nevada as a fitting living memorial when the cataclysmic destruction of their continent ended their civilization so many millenniums ago, just as later the Atlanteans left us reminders of their scientific culture in Egyptian and Mayan pyramids. It was intended as the lofty spiritual heritage for the hermitages of sages, predestined to become a Western Spiritual Center that will herald the rise of a Pacific continent again, now that man has suffered and toiled bringing the progress of culture to encircle the globe from the Pacific shores of Asia westward persistently to the Pacific shores of California again. Notice how man's religious progress and spiritual current travels westward propelled by the sun-after the "Cradle of Civilization" in Central Asia from which the Aryans fostered the ancient Chinese culture, then the Hindu and Buddhist along with the Zoroastrian in Persia, followed by the Greeks and the transforming of the Jews as Christianity spread west and north throughout Europe and now also embraces America in doctrine. Finally, here in the golden west is the melting pot for the purification to obtain the spiritual gold of all our past religious cultures, the new racial heritage gathered with all man's gleanings of knowledge to synthesize the direct path of perfection in God's Government on earth now that the cycle of time is ripe to harvest the Golden Age again. For religious culture, look to the Golden West, and Be Like the Sequoia, the symbol of Everlasting Life and an ever-living tree-creation so appropriately perfected by the Lemurians as our living heritage thru the ages.

VITARIANISM, the LIFE-CONSERVATION-VENERA-TION movement has been God's inner progressive purpose of all true culture. This is the ETERNAL CHRIST Principle that spiritualized man from the beginning of time. Obeying the Life Principle in all things, doing the Creator's Will by preservation of the continuance of His word, to identify with God,-Spirit, Truth and Love,-constantly in our thoughts, actions and being is the Christ Perfection taught as God's Government (or Kingdom), which is the Commandments of Life or Law Divine found universally as the essential teachings of all religions. Each time great civilizations were established, they came with holymen among them who worked for their betterment, but the profaning and disrespect of religion as a means of perpetuating corrupt living, caused the decay and fall of these civilizations as the Life Principle removed westward to a new body of men. Each man is given Life whose Law he must live, but corruption instead of conservation and veneration of this Inner Life Principle brings death to his body as life seeks better vehicles for progress.

1. HUMANITARIAN: The first great Life-Conservation-Veneration Principle that blossoms from man's first spiritual aims. With cannibal habits, whether eating the victims or killing and injuring for pleasure, man cannot conserve himself individually nor collectively in the Law of Being.

2. VEGETARIAN: Studying the lives of great thinkers, saints, and teachers of mankind in all times we find them practicing God's commandment, "Thou shalt not kill" to the extent of vegetarianism. "If a man have a hundred sheep...it is not the will of

your Father in heaven that a single one of these little ones should perish," said the Christ, Jesus who caused Christianity to substitute a bloodless sacrifice at the altar for the former slaughtered offerings. If Christianity could get back to the vegetarian principles of the saints and early followers, in cooperation with the non-violence and vegetarian doctrine of Buddhists and Brahmins, the world would be unanimously vegetarian and with universal abolition of bloodshed the earth would have true Peace. Vegetarians point out their solution of famines threaten mankind showing that if land is used for grains instead of for meat production there is a 15 to 20 times greater yield.

3. VITARIAN: The revolutionary consideration presented to advanced thinkers today after abstinence from killing other men and killing animals, is the abstinence from man's slow suicide. In the Christ-Life-Principle without sin, "death shall be no more." Holymen have long advocated strict continence knowing that human seed waste prevents spirituality, and the Vitarian teaching reveals pollutions, menstruation or any loss of seed to be the beginning of degeneration. The reproductive cells called an "embryonic tumor" by a medical doctor for being intermediate between growth and tumors of age, we have found to be caused by the diet of superfluous albumins and reproductive substance that abounds in the granivorous. The elimination of this parasitic tumorous growth of reproductive cells that degenerate man, comes thru eliminating nuts, grains and other seeds, using only fruits and herbs which was the original God-Given dietetic law which gave man nearly a millennium of life as happened with Methuselah, or immortality without death as the case of Methuselah's father, Henoch, who was translated without dying already at 365 years, to mortal flesh ascending into spiritual absorption in Perfection. Vegetarianism often includes use of dairy foods still requiring the enslaving of animals and gaining second-hand food requiring still the greater acreage for pastures. Vitarianism emphasizes avoiding the by-products obtained by slaughter such as leather, and also advocates live or Vita-foods rather than typical abundance of morbid matter taken as food by even vegetarians. Moreover, Vitarianism claims the root cause of famines and need, is seen in countries that are vegetarian such as India which are the very site of famines, and is because they live

on a granivorous vegetarian diet which causes the outstanding increase in the birth rate compared to other nations, creating the over-population, and makes necessary the growing of seed crops, especially grains, which deplete the soil fertility rapidly compared to fruit trees that replenish own losses in humus and go deeper for added minerals besides hold the moisture, and prevent erosion caused by the cultivation of grains, legumes, seeds, etc., which require the plowing and loosening of soil that is soon wasted away by washing. Vitarianism aims for Life Conservation by reforestation with fruit trees rather than defor-estation by soil depleting crops.

4. FRUITARIAN: The ideal of Vitarians is to have all their food from fruit trees, eliminating yearly the planting and cultivation between the trees before fruit is born, in their gardens. Certainly fruits are more delicious, freer of earthy qualities, purifying the body, promoting intense spiritual power. However, as the Bible legend goes, man is forbidden the use of the fruit of a certain tree, which is the nut tree, whose fruit has degenerated leaving only the seed (from the peach, apricot, etc., degenerated the almond). Because of the ignorance of this factor, fruitarianism has not proven more successful, because raw nuts as well as any raw seeds are the very potent human seed activator and the tumorous sex growth thus created wastes away the other tissue of the body (teeth, nerves, brain cells) which give character and elements to the human seed. When I say, "Nuts make you nutty" this is not a mere joke, but a lamentable fact I have observed from experimenters, the nutarians and seed diet advocates fast losing potency and taking on the "not-responsible person" psychosis, with continual mental inconsistency being often psychic-dream world victims. Man desires the Paradise of Pleasure, Eden, but the Flaming Sword cuts off his attempt of any approach if he will not abstain from the forbidden food, consuming seed for pleasure till death rules.

5. BREATHARIAN: The Oriental "Yoga" technique of breathing is used to take in greater quantities of ordinary dense air which contains considerable water condensed in the body using a special compressing full breath, absorbing into the lungs and even the stomach solar energy, just as we utilize vitamins electrically and not chemically, and the organic life in the dense

jungle air. The organic 5. BREATHARIAN: The Oriental "Yoga" technique of breathing is used to take in greater quantities of ordinary dense air which contains considerable water condensed in the body using a special compressing full breath, absorbing into the lungs and even the stomach solar energy, just as we utilize vitamins electrically and not chemically, and the organic life in the dense jungle air. The organic and gaseous materials thus concentrated are thus equal to the amount of substances found in an ordinary fruit diet but gas is the medium of suspension rather than water. The Purification of the body comes entirely by burning or oxidation. Though of equal merit in some ways it is not so accessible to Westerners nor fitting into the Order of the Aquarian Age of the present.

6. AQUARIAN: The new "Aquarian Age" revelation in the Western "Aquarian" or Christian Natural Technique is the Spontaneous Path to the realization of giving up eating which consists in body purification by cleansing by water (aqua), balance and sublimation of male and female currents of energy, and ecstatic spiritual contemplation. The "Aquarian" regimen using tinctured water, coordinated with ecstatic breath of contemplatives and a number of other factors is now being perfected by the writer to make the transition and mastery practical for advanced disciples in general. Mountain hermitages with coniferous trees will be sought for the practice to obtain ozone in more rarefied air rather than lowlands or the jungle where the heavier oxygen is given off as a by-product of luxuriant trees and vegetation.

7. HELIOARIAN: Eventually, the return to the original perfection by complete purification by ozone to eliminate the mortal "clay" or elements that keep one earth-bound by gravity to achieve the ascension into complete absorption by the Supreme Infinite Spirit, will enable one to depend solely on a solar sustenance. This is the Goal in Immortalism, Eternal Youth Life continued to a complete cycle of earth experience and Omniscience, to transcend death by absorption or direct resurrection into Spiritual Essence. The Great Teachers, most notably Christ, achieved this lofty mission but often it may result men will say more "he was seen no more" having ascended from the pinnacle or snows of some super-attitude to

Eternity.

AQUARIAN TINCTURE ANALYSIS

The following Chart (based on Sherman's analysis) is to be used as a beginner's guide for the preparation of tinctured wash water for constant inner baptism of the alimentary canal from less than assimilable quantities of acid fruit juice. Fruits to be selected are of no value if they do not contain enough acid and too much readily assimilable nourishment so as to activate the digestive juices giving the return of hunger on the Aquarian perpetual fast. The mention of 1% nutritionally valued tincture with 99% water, does not mean any of it is to be assimilable, and it will be found that the acid unripe oranges and grapefruit (often marketed without a full sugar quota), besides other uncooked characteristically acid fruit juices can be used one-third to nearly one-half glass of juice with each full glass of flavored water (with no sweetener), and taken copiously not only clean out the whole digestive tract and intestines with its acid-liquid mucous-solvent detergent but also prevent complete assimilation of the water by the kidneys, providing a pint or more of water to wash the intestines and colon in natural direction rather than by water forced up backwards artificially by enemas or colonics. If obtainable, Distilled Water is to preferred to avoid the calcareous inorganic materials in ordinary earth water (springs, etc.) Experience rather than analysis of select fruit nutritionally, will show how to avoid assimilable kinds and amount of fruit juice to give return to hunger, and what is best to purge and baptize the human body to become an immaculate temple of the Living God throughout.

| % OF: | WATER | PROTEIN | FAT | CARBO | ASH | CALS/lb. | Comment |
|---|---|---|---|---|---|---|---|
| Apple juice | 87.1% | 0.1% | 2.5% | | 0.25 | 230 | good from tart apples |
| Grapefruit juice | 89.3% | 0.4% | 0.1% | 9.8% | 0.4% | 190 | good |
| Grape juice | 80.7% | 0.4% | | 18.5% | 0.39 | 345 | Tart kinds better |
| Orange juice | 85.7% | 0.6% | | 13.1 | 0.58 | 250 | Avoid ripe and sweet |
| Peach juice | 86.5% | 0.2% | | 12.8 | 0.5 | 235 | |
| Pineapple juice | 85.3% | 0.3% | 0.3% | 12.8% | 0.4% | 272 | Good unsweetened |
| Strawberry juice | 94.2% | .2% | | 5.1% | 0.45 | 95 | Excellent |
| Tomato juice canned | 94.0 | 1.0 | 0.1 | 3.6 | 0.9 | 97 | Excellent |

## WHOLE FOODS

| % OF: | WATER | PROTEIN | FAT | CARBO | ASH | CALS/lb. | Comment |
|---|---|---|---|---|---|---|---|
| Cucumber | 96.1 | 0.7 | 0.1 | 2.7 | .44 | 65 | Excellent w. tom. juice |
| Watermelon | 92.1 | 0.5 | 0.2 | 6.9 | 0.27 | 190 | Nature's Distilled H2O |
| Tomatoes fresh | 94.1 | 1.0 | 0.3 | 4.0 | 0.57 | 105 | Excellent fresh juice |
| Figs | 78.0% | 1.4 | 0.4 | 19.6 | 0.64 | 395 | Sweetener; sour juice |
| Raisins seedless | 17.0 | 2.6 | 0.2 | 80.2 | 1.6 | | Sweetener for teas etc. |

% OF:WATER  PROTEIN  FAT  CARBO ASH  CALS/lb. Comment

| | WATER | PROTEIN | FAT | CARBO | ASH | CALS/lb. | Comment |
|---|---|---|---|---|---|---|---|
| Sorghum or sorgo | | 2.4 | | 63.0 | | 1180 | Sweetener for teas |

HERBS

| | WATER | PROTEIN | FAT | CARBO | ASH | CALS/lb. | Comment |
|---|---|---|---|---|---|---|---|
| Beets | 87.6 | 1.6 | 0.1 | 9.6 | 1.11 | 120 | Toxic oxalic acid |
| Cabbage white | 92.4 | 1.4 | 0.2 | 5.3 | 0.75 | 130 | Poor flavorer |
| Cabbage curly | 87.3 | 4.1 | 0.6 | 6.2 | 1.8 | 211 | Much protein |
| Celery | 93.7 | 1.3 | 0.2 | 3.7 | 1.08 | 100 | Good flavorer in tom. |
| Chard, leaf | 91.0 | 2.6 | 0.4 | 4.8 | 1.2 | 150 | Oxalic toxic, pasty |
| Dandelion | 85.8 | 2.7 | 0.7 | 8.8 | 0.95 | 235 | Alkalizer flavoring |
| Kale | 86.6 | 3.9 | 0.6 | 7.2 | 1.7 | 225 | Protein. |
| Lettuce | 94.8 | 1.2 | 0.2 | 2.9 | 0.91 | 85 | Soporiferous lactucar. |
| Mustard | 92.2 | 2.3 | 0.3 | 4.0 | 1.21 | 125 | Irritating oil of mustard |
| Nettles | 82.4 | 5.5 | 0.7 | 9.1 | 2.3 | 295 | High protein, pasty |
| Watercress | 93.9 | 1.7 | 0.3 | 3.3 | 1.09 | 105 | Kidney irritant |

The herbs or vegetables given in latter part of the Chart are not recommended but given for comparisons and objections, not being purifying, contain nourishment we want to avoid now but in an emergency may be tried. Herbs we recommend for flavoring tomato water were parsley, celery, basil, etc., and for teas,-spearmint, chamomile, peppermint, etc. The Aroma and flavoring without nutrition is sought to aid the drinking of a great amount of water, more or less a gallon. To figure out Percent of supposed nutrition in a juice, add up the Protein, fat, carbohydrate and ash percents which, for example, are 5.6% in tomato juice meaning that by using little over four parts water and one part juice (one to five) your tinctured water has a 1% amount of supposed nutritional value diluted in 99% water. Your writer will appreciate the experiences of others on various juices used on tinctured water regimen, even if they use the new Non-eating Technique just as cleansing fast is employed ordinarily. It will take more experience, of a number of Vitarians and over a period of time to determine any more definite rules than now given. Abstaining from what nourishes man in his mortality and death, we can nourish completely from real substance, Immortal and Omnipotent, the Living Bread of Christ. May you seek to live "by every word of God"!

LESSON XXI

PREFACE TO A COSMIC UNIVERSAL BIBLE

The constantly agitated multitudes are involved in the futility of seeking worldly Peace, while each nation or faith remains isolated, each in their own knowledge and understanding of its own religious scriptures, history, culture and traditions; all of which may condemn others to the point of intolerant prohibition in the study and presentation of facts universally. There is much more knowledge than is recorded in a single Holy Scripture of any people. Too much of the earth's population would limit its information to what the political bosses feed them with in the newspapers, what they are freely given in sales catalogs, or segregated into by some sectarian religious mission. The minds of men have been patterned and conditioned by their earliest and innermost impressions, and too often while they open themselves willingly to new fields in worldly knowledge and science, spiritually they refuse to broaden their vision.

Why should our 745 million Christians live subject to the traditions, precepts, and religious doctrine of the early prophets of the remaining 14 million Jews? Willingly we swallow the Old Testament History as the Word of God, God's Commandments and laws and undeniable Truth from a sect or small group, one fifty third part of the Christian populations, whose racial heritage the vast majority do not share for being of Caucasian or Aryan descent, while we refuse in the average Christian denomination to accept or even associate the ancient wisdom teachings and prophets of the Aryan race accepted by the 800 million of the Brahmin-Buddhist world (which exceeds our Christian population), as Divine or even profitable for investigation? Briefly, we are not trying to give out an anti-semitic or hate-Jews propaganda, willing to return love for their spitting on and massacre of Christ and Christian besides continued profanity, any more than we care to dwell on the profaning of Christian teachings by the Koran and the Mohammedans, but why worship according to Old Testament Theology, while ignoring and intolerant to Oriental Theology which accepts the Divinity of Christ, lives by the commandments of Jesus and prophesied the coming of Christ also in their teachings? Is this all-loving and democratic? What right have we Westerners to sit back and label the rest "Pagan, idolaters, and heathens", claiming the Judo-Christian Bible as the oracle of Truth, beyond which no other Verities can exist?

The Jewish History in the Old Testament is a mere fraction of man's history on earth, which began thousands of years before Adam, with marvels far beyond the story of the Hebrew nation. The millions of Christians besides Jews have accepted this as all and only! The Jewish Bible marks off the earth as a mere 4 or 6 thousand years old in its history of man, while the Hindu "Bhagavad Gita" of their Bible has existed over 5 thousand years, besides the inaccessible stone records in the Himalayas giving the "record of man through the ages" mapping the world in the days of Lemuria, and later the history and sinking of Atlantis, giving us history over 70,000 years old. James Churchward, famous archeologist, whose books ("Lost

Continent of Mu" etc.) are to be had at the Public Libraries, mastered the Lemurian language, and with the evidence of stone records (which cannot change by recopying and trans- lating) and the wondrous cities, temples and highways found in various parts of the Pacific not sub-merged with the conti- nent's sinking that science accepts as irrefutable evidence of a superior civilization, besides the mythical traditions of peoples the world over on the "Golden Age", show us that MUCH is left out between Chapter I and II in Genesis. First we are told that man, which is later referred to as the "sons of god", were first created in the Image of God and "male and female, He created them," meaning the first men were hermaphrodites or bisexual not needing to mate or reproduce, and then Moses tells how Adam, a member of the Perfect people, fell and was expelled from Paradise to go live somewhere in Atlantis with his wife, Eve. Moses gives the moral history of man, how he fell dis- obeying the first law God gave to man forbidding him to eat anything more than fruits and herbs, how some who walked with God in this first law of God lived astounding ages such as Methuselah, and whose father never saw death being trans- lated directly into Supreme Spirit, while others having devel- oped extra-nourishing foods such as wheat for bread, drinking milk, etc., grew into giants in stature from the flesh producing qualities of these foods besides the carnal passion-stimulating attributes causing them to shorten man's life expectancy to 120 years through bestial reproduction rather than the original bisexual propagation and "their heart was bent on evil at all times."

Now the bread-eating man of wondrous physique and great scientific intellect accomplished wonders equal to our world of today, the stone tablets in various places in the Lemu- rian language record the development of atomic airships and weapons with which they caused the destruction of Atlantis in explosions till it sank under the Atlantic Ocean, and Moses records this as the Great Flood that came from God's dissatis- faction in man. When Noe landed on Mr. Ararat there was no vegetation of any kind on earth for man's food, so God is said to have permitted certain meats if the blood was not used, or shall we say his conscience bothered him less about killing now. Their hearts hardened by killing animals and with animal properties in their veins, they were easily led into becoming a warring nation.

There is a general pattern through which all religions have been exploited to profanely "religionize" the world. Realizing that religion touches the innermost convictions of men it has been exploited as a "shield" to inspire evil deeds of men, because lost in their lower sensual seekings they do not think, letting their leaders lead them to and into slaughter like helpless sheep merely because they use the Holy Names and Word of God in their vicious battle cry. Here we have the Jews coming out of Egypt saying they were led by a cruel God in His will to march north to kill, rape and steal cities of all who opposed them preaching a moral code against their methods. Later their prophets foretold the coming of a Messiah to become King of the Jews, but when He did appear they rejected Him, perhaps for being from a Gentile people like the rest of the Galileans though they did patronize the Jewish religion. But the new covenant of a compassionate God, Christ taught, ordering the giving up of the bloody sacrifice of animals, demanding the return of love for hate, praise for injury, good for evil,-giving His life to exemplify this,-and depreciating the old traditions. Practice of essential religious principles proved itself as the Spiritual Truth for the souls of men, gradually converting the European civilization in doctrine, though again it was used as teaching, not exemplary practice, as the wars that blood-stained the centuries progressed.

Long before the Jewish conquests, all this was enacted by other peoples, besides the Jews, from the Atlantians who survived the sinking of Atlantic and conquested the peaceful white people living in the high Andies in structures of architecture using immense stones in perfect fit besides engineering feats in canals, etc., now unduplicable, and who overcame the white Lemurian people of pre-Mayan times of Mexico. Later the Europeans "Christianized" the Incas and the Mayans, killing all who refused to accept the "merciful Prince of Peace" peddled by the pirates' priests. And so far, we have only spoken about the origin of the Jewish race from Atlantis, but let us get back before all this to the Aryan descendents of Lemuria who can be accounted for, the remains of cities over a 100,000 years old in the Gobi desert, where tablets have been found in the Lemurian language. Very recent to this Aryan Culture in central Asia, is the setting of the 5,000 year old Bhagavad Gita which we might parallel in ways to a Hindu "Old Testament." The Gita comes forth on the plains of India in a bloody battle between the "Pandavas" of the dark people of the south who claimed a spiritual teaching symbolically involved in their conquest, while they conquered the "Kurus," the tribal name of Aryans "inhabiting Central Asia beyond the Himalayas, who migrated with other races into the northwest of the peninsula and with them formed the great people who styled themselves unitedly Arya, or the noble, to distinguish them from the aborigines whom they subdued later." Of the Pandus "Arjuna is horror struck at the idea of committing fratricide by slaying his near relations and throws down his bow and arrows, declaring that he would rather be killed without defending himself than fight against them." But Krishna who styles himself as God counselling him, warns Arjuna of the spirit of cowardice and gives a gospel of non-attachment to action, justifying the bravery in fighting rather than self-sacrificing compassion. From this, Krishna elucidates the Paths of Yoga and brings out the symbology of the battle fought, as the conquest of soul over the ignorance of body senses and mind. Krishna, the warrior spirited God is deified, which with its traditions and rituals, finds approval of the Hindus to this day, just as the Jewish traditions of God-inspired wars remain the doctrine of Jews besides the Christians, and are used as arguments for continuing our present wars, killing, and sins of mankind. Do not think the Gita does not have very profound truth identical or comparable to the Christian Bible, but all the inspiration unfortunately was built on a questionable example as to the teaching of non-violence and pacifism, which the Hindus practice today, based on other spiritual teachings.

Then many centuries later came the Lord Buddha, with his gospel of compassion to all things, demanding the strict observation of the Dharma (the Law) just as the Christ demanded the strict keeping of God's Commandment (or Law) in His teaching. Buddha then rejected the traditional rituals, altar sacrifices, pretenses of hypocritical religious piety Caste or class system and the non-essential practices, but just as Jesus was rejected in his own country, the Buddha also was rejected as the official teaching or faith in India, though his gospel became the popular belief to the north in Tibet, China, besides the greatest philosophical foundation of Asia's spirituality in general. The Buddha purged the concept of Divinity from all human attributes, to the extent that western missionaries often try to confuse it with atheism since their lofty reference to a transcendent Supreme Spirit of Omniscience, Super-conceptional Truth and Peace Profound, does not fit under the attributes the primitive war-lords gave to their man-conceived god of early Judaism. Buddhism was not rejected, however, in the sense Christianity is rejected by the Jews, but rather the teachings of Buddhas became a part of certain parts of the Hindu religion, which by the way does not have an official "One and Only Avatar or Saviour" allowing also Christ as a teacher even, so that we have Buddhist Yogis, and in China the teachings of Buddha are supplemented by those of Confucius and Lao Tze. The two, including the branches of later philosophies, characterize a Brahmin-Buddhist Doctrine just as united essentially, if not more so, as all the various Christian denominations and more than Christianity's equal in democratic considerations, of acceptance, without priest and preacher pressure types of conversion, literature and radio monopoly to speak of, if at all.

However, this does not mean practice of absolute non-violence throughout eastern Asia, -hardly is it a solid front in India,-and Buddhist nations were corrupted from the absolute non-killing, permitting animal slaughter under ritual, and once men are hardened by the substance of beasts in their own blood, they willingly commit bloodshed so that we have the atrocious happenings in China, Indo-China, Japan and Korea. The example of Christianity is just too feeble and the great proof that claiming a religion has given people nothing. Christ being practical and effective in practice only. The Eastern Buddhist World and Western Christian World are realizing that the real Spiritual Principle of Truth is in the PRACTICE OF COMPASSIONATE LOVE as SUPREME WISDOM, esteeming non-violence and selfless sacrifice as practical spiritual power, rather than either confusing intellectual battles or bloody "religious" wars as practiced in the tribal uncultured primitive doctrines of our society and early man.

On this doing of the LAW in the LIGHT of LOVE in this LIFE Everlasting of the Spiritual Realm, besides the Peace and Well Being of all beings on earth now, and basis of the gospels of both Christ and Buddha. The conquest of the world for these principles of Spirituality will come only thru strict exemplification, and the challenge is whether your are able to become Emancipated to live wholly on the Spiritual plane in all practicality. Otherwise in the ways of the world, slave and tool to an everlasting contagion doing evil works to promote good in theory, nothing is ever accomplished as mankind flirts with extinction this very day. The only practical religion, the only practical spirituality for anyone is not mental religion based on precepts in theories of doctrines. Every minute the mind changes its color, tone and shape, and this can be no firm foundation to build the living Temple of God which instead is the body involving a manner of life which takes years of discipline to change permanently, getting our "faith into our bones" as well as being and soul. The down to earth practical Truth, religion or spirituality has to be a physical religion in practice also, as well as thus seeking completion on all planes. Otherwise Peace is only a slogan for our wars, philanthropy the motive of more exploitation of laborers and religion the front for campaigns of separation, hate, confusion and human weak-morals. The world is also getting too specialized. History of war, patriotism and military training are taught in schools and colleges as compulsory needs, but religion, if at all, comes separately, independent in Sunday School as though not connected with life's necessities. We need a live religion, to live it on earth balanced in everyday lives and make it equally everyday child-training to cultivate the qualities that give man Peace. Of course, here again the need of a democratic Universal Scripture accepted by all parts of the world, and the education of teachers in Comparative Religions so they will know the basic essential teachings of all religions, is seen.

A hating condemnation of anything, including religion, race, way of sustenance, etc., shows a residue of the same weakness within accuser's own makeup, and complete experience is shown by indifference or equal-view in the victorious soul. A recently converted vegetarian in his enthusiasm would forcefully take the meat away from all while his body "has been built" from meat and the cells cry for old meat stimulants creating his haughty indignation and unpeace toward others who might be ready to follow him, if his actions of loving compassion proved himself. The same is true of the white race superiority advocate since Grace or Cosmic Law often gives the fairest of complexions and features to the ignorant and immoral so they may learn the vanity and suffering in losing physical power and respect, while often in our darker brothers have appeared teachers of High Spirituality that God chose the humility of appearance,-greater than color, vain beauty of impressive features-to guard His deep wisdom. Religion is slandered by those, who like her members, refuse to live by the doctrines.

Just as DIVINE LIFE CONSERVATION is the inner "mystery" or purpose that the seeming life necessity of eating or sustenance contributes to man's spiritual evolution, DIVINE LIFE VENERATION is the inner mystery or purpose that the seeming or contradictory necessity of education or culture contributes to man's spiritual development. Education, culture or civilization embrace the extremes of virtue and evil, the heavenward path and the wide road to oblivion of mankind! The highest spiritual culture has been conserved in apostolic order in scriptures, teachings and techniques of spiritual development through our Holy Orders of religions dedicated to the absolute devotion to God throughout the ages by Holymen. These Holymen who renounce the world to fully dedicate their lives to the spiritual development through our Holy Orders of religions dedicated to the absolute devotion to God throughout the ages by Holymen. These Holymen who renounce the world to fully dedicate their lives to the spiritual welfare of mankind, purity of body and mind, non-attachment to worldly pleasures and great discipline,-and thus are called ascetics, monks, masters, hermits, devotees, religious prophets, etc.,-have carried the sacred wisdom not only by conserving the records from man's Golden Age in Lemuria, but by practice have kept them living in our hearts by this select group of God's elect. Like the records of most ancient wisdom from Lemuria, men live these principles of the Ancient Order in example, giving mankind its contact with the first Son of God that dwell in a perfect race, and later was Revived in yoga teachings and its ascetic orders. Revitalized by Buddha and his holy orders and finally resurrected in Christ and Christian orders of saints. The teachings would have been worthless and scoffed at as primitive superstition, etc., if the living proof in men had not remained with men always, and the exemplification of such revolutionary principles would have been sheer insanity in the minds of men, had not the record of most ancient religious attainment required this. How else would you or anyone else be able to share of the Supreme Treasure, the Immortal Heritage of all Ages, if it were not for education so as to get the living truth in a humanly recognizable form? And it is one thing to see a saint, an ascetic live the renunciation for which the ignorant ridicule him for giving up the worldly pleasures they love, and an equally inadequate condition to read religious scriptures or deep philosophy without seeing its practicality lived in men in exemplary reason and worth.

Now as to the source that brought the Ancient Sacred Order to Christianity from the East, there is much convincing evidence, though various authors will seek to accredit their own source of interest for the Christ. The scriptures make HIM "Orient on High", who was heralded by the wise men from the East at his birth (just as Buddhas are traditionally) besides given guidance for his protection throughout his life, and who literally translated the oriental science of Yoga or "yoke" he described sweet light besides philosophic truths of the Enlightened ones or Buddhas for which He is known as the Light of the World. Just as St. Augustine said, "The Christian Religion really was known to the Ancients, nor was it wanting at any time from the beginning of the human race, until the time when Christ came into the flesh, most religious leaders have felt the influence of the Christ Principle as the Eternal Truth of religion that has accompanied the progress of culture in the Christian people or race as it came westward to encircle the globe from the origin in paradise of the Pacific Continent. Prominent is the consideration that Jesus was an Essene. Prof. E. B. Szekely, who has translated the "Essene Gospel of John" from the Aramaic tongue from manuscripts that are filed under record number 156-P in the Vatican library in Rome, says in his introduction of the scripture: The Essenes created the greatest synthesis of religions, philosophies, and sciences of human history on the basis of Organic Unity of the Hebrew, Egyptian,

Greek, Persian, Babylonian and Hindu Cultures. Is not this wonderful harmonious synthesis an inspiration to us for a unificative reconciliation of all the values of the universal culture in an optimum and omnilateral contemporary synthesis? Is not the basic Essene principle of active love (taught by the Essene Prophets and by the greatest Essenes, John the Baptist, Jesus the Christ, and John the Beloved), the eternal foundation of all religions and ethics? Never before has suffering Humanity faced such a great need for a modern Essene Renaissance than at the present. "Now the first copies of the Christian Scriptures of the first century were scrolls circulated among the Christians, the first ones being made by Matthew who is believed to have recorded the history of Jesus as he saw it happen, while Mark and Luke copied facts from Matthew adding new findings from records made by other witnesses, while John, being the Master's favorite, was asked to study the other scrolls and give material not given in Matthew, revised by Mark and Luke in their gospels, both of which never saw Jesus but like Paul whom they carried books for and attended on his journeys, were not contemporaries of Jesus. Thus MOST of the NEW TESTAMENT is written by men who never saw Jesus from the conversion of Paul thru Grace of the Holy Spirit, thru a rapturous vision of Christ, which by the way was the means of conversion to Christ of your writer through Grace prior to which he was completely unread in Christian Bible texts. So the true story and inner teachings of Jesus, from eye-witness accounts are to be found with Matthew written in Aramaic before 42 A.D. and John, Beloved disciple of Christ, whom most accept as having shared more of the hidden experiences of their Master.

Debaters see only one side of a question,-their own side. To prove their side they put on blinders incapable of seeing anything else. This is the cause of our modern educated illiteracy, with sects and denominations preaching one little doctrine they wish to recognize only, besides the specialization in all fields of promotion that seeks to confusingly battle for the one side of the perspective they see.

Now let us study another source in uncommon knowledge about Jesus not found in the popular version of the Bible.

The "Peshitta" or Eastern Text" of the New Testament, was composed of scrolls of Matthew, who wrote 10 or 15 years after the Crucifixion giving gospel on Aramaic before Paul's conversion, from which Paul preached and gave his commentaries, with the addition of the writings of John, gave us the complete Aramaic compilation in 150 A.D. George Lamsa, who gave us the English translation direct from the Aramaic text, says: "The Ecclesiastical authorities of all the Christian churches in the Near East, the Ancient Church of the East, the Monophysites, and Maronite Roman Catholics believe that the New Testament and the liturgies were introduced into the churches of Syria and Mesopotamia by the Apostles. They all believe that Christianity started from the East, that Easterners were the first converts and that their churches were established first. "There is no mention of any translation of the New Testament being made into Aramaic in the Catholic Church councils of third and fourth centuries, and after the Greek version from which later they translated the Latin "Vulgate," till the Rheims (1582) and Douay (1610) versions of the Catholics, beside the King James Version made less than three and a half centuries ago, our western world has had no text on the gospel of Jesus, while the Eastern Church has had its Bible and services conducted in the Aramaic tongue native to them since the Master Jesus sent 70 disciples to Mesopotamia to preach and the Apostles compiled the Eastern text. Lamsa brings out many astounding facts about the original gospel in Aramaic, but since our interest is relating to whether Jesus was an Essene, this is what he says: "The doctrine of celibacy and abstinence from wine, meat and certain foods were introduced by the Essenes, Sabians, and members of other ancient cults who had embraced Christianity. Some went so far in their asceticism that they abstained from eating cultivated plants and vegetables. Their doctrines were supposed to have been based on God's commands concerning food as found in Genesis. (Gen. 1:29) They blamed the fall of man and his short life upon his departure from this command. Many of these people were found in Syria and Asia Minor. Some believers in these ancient cults are still to be found in the East. Paul denounced these doctrines as alien to the Scriptures and not founded on the truth of Jesus Christ (See Rom. 14:2, I Time. 4:3, etc.) He claims there are some 10,000 Sabians in Iraq who follow the

Baptism of John Baptist in teaching as well as believe in Jesus. But Lamsa goes on to classify Jesus as a "Nazarite", who are identified by their long hair as a mark of their consecration to God, which are among the "Kadishey", translated "saints" in our Bible including priests, Nazarites and others, who ministered in the temple and were supported by offerings. Moreover, Jesus, being a Galilean, was not a Jew, since Galileans were Gentiles brought over from Assyria and Persia (See IV Kings 17) in the time of the Zoroastrian age known for the "Sun-worship", which the Assyrians called "Shamash" and is known in Persian as Mazda, and their people are the Aryans migrated from Central Asia. The distinction Gentile refers to gentle, or noble and good birth in that region and India translated "Aryan" just as we say gentlemanly. The Jews were in turn taken out of Galilee and transplanted in Assyria and Persia by their King, so that the genealogy of Jesus that was not in original Aramaic scrolls but later added gives 28 generations in Matthew while over 40 generations are given in Luke and must be attributed to fanciful guesswork besides erroneous as to Jewish origin. The Jews resented a Galilean, who they looked upon as Gentiles in spite of their Synagogue education, to be called " King of the Jews", and they knew Jesus' disciples who were Galileans by their foreign accent in Jerusalem. Jesus was in truth a "priest forever after the order of Melchisedec," and Melchisedec is also of Mesopotamian-Aryan origin. King of Salem means of Peace and Righteousness, which were scripturally attributed to Jesus, who carried forth the ANCIENT ARYAN ORDER from "Mu" or Lemuria westward, and whose priests were ordained by God so that Christ's priesthood does not stem to the Jewish priesthood that had to be from the house of Aaron and not of homeless poor like Jesus.

What has made the traditions and precepts on religious doctrine of the Jews the heritage of our Aryan or Caucasian peoples? Haven't the Aryans had Prophets of God and Scriptures from God? Why all the preaching in the Christian's name on Israel as to the "saved"? Shouldn't we impartially broaden our study instead of being only partial to the records of traditional heritage of the Jews in millenniums of ignorant plunders and violations of a law they couldn't keep themselves, but attribute of God and Christians-in-their-blinders take as the only holy thing on earth? Instead of letting the religious ministers of His day push Him around by claiming their Scripture was the "word of God" to accuse Him as a sinner, Jesus rebelled as should you and I, and pointed out what was of God and what was the dead word of dead men. The gospel of Jesus taught how the scriptural "letter killeth", while Christ was the very Life Eternal, that the bloody sacrifices of altar ritual taking the Life of sheep, turtles, etc., for man's sins was absolutely vain and abhorrable to God asking the priests of the temples to transform it to commemorating Christ or Life by Conservation taking fruit juices and fasting and by Veneration giving one's self wholly to God, through which He showed Life indestructible, resurrecting after a shameless mob murder. This is the inner baptism of fasting on water cleansing of body and Prayer cleansing of mind that John of the Inner Circle of Teaching brought out in his Essene gospel, as well as the Gospel we have on birth for water and Holy Spirit (John 3:5), instead of flesh, meat or bread which perisheth, for overcoming hunger, want and death to have Life Everlasting. (John 3:6;6:27,35,52,58)! John Beloved, presented his message like Jesus in the loving Gentile-noble-Aryan manner of the Galileans, while the former persecutor newly converted Jew, Paul, ambitiously aggressive even for his new cause with his aids Mark and Luke, worked in the Baptism of Blood, saving by grace not works ideal that our Christianity has labored in during 19 centuries and monopolize the New Testament. The Spirit of Truth reveals after centuries of blood baptizing, wars and martyrs and mere belief-claiming Christians that Grace is in those who live from being born again for water and Spirit (cells not built of food), "that doth truth, cometh to the light, that his works may be made manifest, because they are done by God." This is the VITA (life) ARYAN (Noble, gentle) message of VITARIANISM, for the Coming Age, Kingdom or Order now at hand declaring Peace to all nations by works in a religion of Love.

Jesus Christ manifested the "Light of the World" by omnisciently combining the teachings of Loving Compassion and Transcendent Wisdom given by the "Light of Asia" (Buddha) with deep re-"search (of) the Scriptures" of Jewish doctrine which often contained truths given by the prophets, but thrashing out the tradition, customs, and precepts of men. Heralded the "Orient from on High" and mocked "King of the Jews", in a first price of penance told us he would not bring men peace, but war, explained the great conflict of lower self and Higher Self of man symbolically portrayed in the Bhagavad Gita. Failing to grasp renunciation of all for Christ, this very day has our warriors at arms, while in the Pulpits the preachers spread "religious venom" because of traditional sayings connected with religious dogma, rather than getting to essentials. Here both Jews and Gentiles are at fault they cannot bear to have their traditions, customs and worldly knowledge rejected. Very few Aryans or Jews have been truly holy enough to bear insult with praise, injury with forgiveness.

Jesus wanted men to see the ESSENTIALS, and went so far as to weed out tradition from the Ten Commandments, which traditional laws contradicted, nor was anyone able to obey them all. The Jews would hold up "parent honor", "adultery", etc., for excuses to kill. Jesus affirmed "Thou shalt not kill" but contradicted the fourth commandment in his requirements of disciples to "hate" or renounce the love of father and mother besides relations, for which people first motivate killing as an act of protecting them as a virtue. Rather, we should Honor the Father of all by calling no man father on earth. For the VITAL "Commandment of God", Christ affirmed only to necessary, that we love God above all in all, and that we love one another, which includes not killing, committing adultery, stealing, bearing false witness and desiring neighbor's possessions, all of which are taught by Jews, Mohammedans, Brahmins, Buddhists, Taoists, etc.,-but special attachment to parents, Jesus exposed well, besides the Jewish Sabbath law.

From the beginning of time, under symbols representing the Eternal Christ-Creator in the sun as the "LIGHT of the world" of Zoroastrians and Incas; in the multiple-formed unformed Brahman, Cause and Creator of all "LIFE" of the Hindus; in the phenomena and concept transcending illumined Buddha emanating all compassionate "LOVE" to all Beings of Buddhists; in the spontaneous selfless Tao as the heart-known "LAW" of the Taoists; and again totally synthesized in Christ-Crucified of the crucifix as the Supreme Light

of the World, Supreme Abundance of Life, Supreme Sacrifice
in life-giving Love for mankind, and the Supreme fulfilling of
the Law,-The LIGHT IN A LIFE OF LOVE,-mankind has wor-
shipped in a "Friends Quaker like" silence peacefully as the
altar incense sweetened and illumined the heart into Love,
God-Oneness, at the temples. Yet today in northern America
with its Atom flash and thunder, the pulpits are filled with those
who likewise thunder in Protestant vehemence with blinding
Old Covenant statutes, accusing all but their sect as heathens,
idolaters and pagans in the out-dated tribal tradition of Juda!
The Old Law perfected nothing, it was the tribal law of the
Order of Aaron but the Christians are to be after the Order of
Melchisedech of the Eastern Peace Kingdom, not of Jewish
genealogy or law. (Heb. 7) And the laws of the perfected Christian Order are written in the hearts and minds of all who seek,
be they Christians, Buddhists, Hindus, or the rest, (Heb. 8;
Jere. 31) for scriptures do not give life to laws. The letter killeth
but Christ-within, spirit quickeneth or vivifies.

We do not know the Sabbath day by a heart quickening
Spirit, like we know sin in wronging our brethren. This being
a calendar calculation and tradition we would not know of if it
were not for Jews. Jesus said in vain do they worship teaching the commandments and doctrines of men (Matt. 15;9)
as God's commandments, and emphatically said the "Sabbath was made for man, not man for the Sabbath." We are
not made thus responsible "for the Sabbath," any more than
we should honor "any man on earth", by calling him "father",
He affirmed because in Christ the "son of man is Lord of the
Sabbath," and we live in the Seventh Day of the Lord, here
and now, in Christ's law for disciples which forbids "laboring for
meat" on any day, commanding renunciation of worldly pursuits, desiring nor seeking "what we shall eat," clothes, wives,
children, or possessions.

Science has shown the "days" of Genesis are periods
or ages as confirmed in Gen. 2:4 "These are the generations...
In the day the Lord God created "showing generations in the
day Adam was created as well as elsewhere a day is a thousand years with God. In the Seventh Day of Creation, God
rested, gave up all his work and ceased to create new things,

just as in this Day of our Lord Christ's Kingdom at hand we should give up our worldly pursuits, in the Holy Life of renunciation. This Sabbath Day of Peace and Prayer of the Heaven-Kingdom of Christ in the Cessation from worldly activity is the meaning of Buddha's "Nirvana" sought in his religious orders of renunciation as well as "Mundaka Upanishad" Hindu teaching of renunciation of action for worldly gain in their Sannyasa orders of Yogis. Jesus did not "observe times" including the Sabbath, saying one should do good works on the Sabbath as well as any day. The Old Covenant accused Jesus of violation of the Ten Commandments, equal to one who kills, steals, etc.! The Apostle Paul (Acts 20:7) records how Christians observed the Eucharistic feast commemorating Lord's Day resurrection with bread-breaking on the Jewish first day of the week or our Sunday. However, he warns judgment of others by Sabbath Day, festivals or times. (Rom. 14:5; Col. 2:16). Jesus' people being of Aryan stock from regions where sun-worship gave them the Sunday, sun-festivals, sun-rise services, etc., must have carried many of their ways with them, one of which was "Shabatum" or day of bad omen of Babylonia. North European Caucasians have used Calendars traditionally with SEVEN DAY as Sunday on right hand side and the older languages count the days by numbers, as in Anglo-Saxon "Oneday" or Monday (Mono for one in monastic), "Two-day" from A.S. root phonetically Tuesday, while the Seventh day is the Sun-day for worship called Rest-day, Lord's day or the dominical. So Jews and Aryans both worship on the Seventh Day Sabbath of the Lord! But how is it that Aryans and Jews count differently?

The whole controversy came because on Lemuria, "Mu", the week was divided into seven days in all her people, but the Aryans progressed westward with the sun from the Lemurian continent to Central Asia, while God had planted the Garden of Eden in the Paradise of Pacific continent "eastward" so with his downfall Adam was exiled by God to Atlantis, where he propagated his people, but when Atlantis sank in the Great Flood Noe landed in the mountains of Armenia. Thus BECAUSE they came counter-sunwise backward around from the International dateline in the pacific, the Jews lost a day, so that their seventh day or Rest Day "Sabbath" of Paradise or Lemuria is the reason in acceptability and acceptance needs to be the UNANIMOUSLY ACCEPTED LIVING DOCTRINE IN SCRIPTURE OF ALL THE WORLD TODAY! Summarizing this multiple page treatise on a Preface to the new UNIVERSAL BI-BLE in all practicality it can consist in three volumes of Sacred Scripture that contain the essential recognized doctrines of the principal religions embracing the unanimous majority of mankind. Such a selection would also bear witness as a Successful Basic Study for every religious student of Truth. The Christ, Who is the Way, Life and Truth has given universal proof to all of His identity in saying, "Search the Scriptures...they bear witness of me."

The Eternal Christ is the Author of Life in our Christian bible, described as "Brahman" of the Hindus, "Buddhi" (Supreme Intelligence or Truth) of the Buddhists, "Tao" Principle of the Taoist, "Ahura Mazda" of the Zoroastrians, etc. If we take the new Covenant of Christ and compare it not only with the rest of the Christian "Holy Bible" (majority accepted Catholic Douay-Rheims Version), but with the main scriptures of the other successful religions, taking for instance the "Buddhist Bible" (Goddard Version with "Tao-Teh-Ching" and other Chinese and Tibetan Sources), and the "Hindu bible" (compiled from Sivananda Versions of the "Bhagavad Gita" and "Principle Upanishads", -we have the essentially identical and true synthesis of the "Word of God" to man. However, the gospels of Hindu and Buddhist Bibles shine like the sun compared to one half of the Hebrew history of wars, exemplification of sins, etc., recorded in the Old Testament, because they give the Noble Path of Renunciation of the World for Spiritual Pursuits, teaching of God-Principle rather than traditions of forefathers, prophets and a human-styled materialistic God. Self-Discipline rather than disciplining others, Infinite compassion or Love for all beings rather than violence, anger and hate, also found in the Sublime Teachings of Christ. The effort here within is impersonal not wishing to defend nor condemn any group or religion, since all peoples, Jews, Catholics, Protestants, Taoists, Buddhists, Hindus, Mohammedans, etc. have been at some time guilty of war and atrocity, showing a need for a more firmly established doctrine. Why should a Universal Doctrine for world acceptance patronize the text of this small group of

Jews, who spit on Christ and put blasphemy on His gospel, for the great volume of the show, when with the addition of Hindu and Buddhist Bibles, no hate of Christ or other condemnations are made, lauding essentially the same principles Christ taught in moral commandments and spirituality. Moreover, with the addition of Hindu and Buddhist Bibles to the Christian Scriptures we have a UNIVERSAL GOSPEL that embraces the vast majority of mankind on earth today. Not only would we benefit by assurances in Spiritual Truths with the basic Three-in-One Bible, but thus the Message of Christ, with contributions of wisdom for Hebrew sages (Isaiah, Moses, etc.) would be given to the greater part of humanity, now ignorant and otherwise unwilling to open their hearts to Christianity. Continuing intolerance others just laugh at the terrible example of Christians, just as most Christian ministers ridicule all others, all in vain. We cannot ask others to examine our scriptures, without prejudice, if we do not do the same to others. Democratic tolerance in religion would thus be demonstrated.